Medical Anecdotes and

T0258966

Nervous
Laughter

Edited by Professor Merton Sandler

from contributions submitted by members of
the General Practitioner Writers Association
and the readership of the
British Journal of Psychiatry

With illustrations by Bernard Cookson

Radcliffe Medical Press · Oxford

© 1991 Radcliffe Medical Press Ltd
15 Kings Meadow, Ferry Hinksey Road, Oxford OX2 0DP

All rights reserved. No part of this publication may be reproduced,
stored in a retrieval system, or transmitted, in any form or by any means,
electronic, mechanical, photocopying, recording or otherwise without the
prior permission of the copyright owner.

British Library Cataloguing in Publication Data

Nervous laughter. – (Medical anecdotes and humour)
 I.   Sandler, Merton   II. Cookson, Bernard
 III. Series
 610.207

 ISBN 1 870905 80 6

Any reference to products in this book does not imply endorsement by
the editor or authors. Any reference to named, living individuals is
purely coincidental.

Typeset by Advance Typesetting Ltd, Oxford
Printed and bound in Great Britain by Billings, Worcester

Contents

1 Introduction

N*ervous Laughter* is distilled from the third series of writing
competitions run by Radcliffe Medical Press, who appointed me to be both judge and executioner. As in any well-
conducted examination, the candidates were known to me
only by a number (although perusal of *Alimentary, My Dear
Doctor* and *Myocardial Medley*, the two previous volumes in
this series, enabled me to make a pretty shrewd guess at
some identities!).

How did I pick the winners? Entries had to be funny, they
had to be relevant to the competition theme and they had to
be well-written. Well, I managed to fill a book without com-
promising these principles but it was touch and go! Many of
the entries were too respectful, not irreverent enough.
Psychiatrists, I've always thought, are fair game and the
more analytical they get, the easier to puncture their
pretensions – if you stand where I stand! Psychiatric
patients, I agree, are a different matter but, if you approach
the task in a good-natured manner, there's a lot of mileage to
be got from them without descending to bad taste.

Many of the entries came into the curate's egg category,
almost literally so for this extract from the entry sent in by
Dr. Robin Hull.

> Beside us on a table was a large tray of eggs. Without
> warning, the man picked one up, cracked it on my
> forehead and broke it open so that raw egg ran down my
> face, matting beard and fogging spectacles. Trying hard to
> preserve decorum I asked 'Why?'. The patient said 'It
> seemed a good idea' – and added a second omelette to the
> first.
>
> Nearly blind, I struggled to the telephone and dialled 999
> to summon help. An urgent voice demanded 'Which
> service?' and, on hearing my request for police help, asked
> for the number I was calling from. My exasperated
> comment 'I don't know . . . I've got egg on my face'
> produced the further irate question 'Is this a hoax?'. It
> took some moments of explanation before the situation
> was accepted and only a few more before a panda-car

screeched up. The two policemen took one look at their well-known village doctor and collapsed in laughter. Eventually one recovered sufficiently to say 'It suits you, Doc!' But the doctor was not amused since a brand-new suit was apparently ruined. However, the insurance company so enjoyed the story that they endorsed the claim form, 'The yolk was on you' and paid in full.

Schizophrenic behaviour of this kind may be a tease but, according to this gem from Dr. W. C. M. Scott, even depression can be a fun thing:

Her alcoholic father deserted her mother and his children. The mother's despair, remorse and feelings of worthlessness led to her collecting their nightly urine and faeces and cooking them for breakfast.

Amatory dalliance was little in evidence but the whimsical final lines of this submission from Dr. A. Shah may deserve mention:

One day they had looked through one of her father's gardening books and somehow came to 'Hollyhock'. There and then, they decided that this would be Tom's pet name for Mary, as the final sentence in the paragraph was 'does well behind hedges but not so well in beds'.

Aggressive psychopathy seems to be the theme of the poem from Dr. M. A. Launer, of which I liked two stanzas:

They're openin' an 'ospital at Wigan,
To cater for bruises an' knocks.
They thowt it had better be big 'un,
Wi a special department for t'pox.

Quite often they'll pull out a switch blade,
And wave it around your big end.
And if they see even a twitch made
There'll be fillets pushed down the S-bend.

Among the veritable broadside of entries from Dr. J. H. Pitt-Payne, one or two shots landed close to the mark:

Much has been said about psychiatry and the men and women who practice the craft. Apparently, they have gone down deeper, stayed down longer, and come up dirtier than any of their medical colleagues. Make no mistake, they all started out in life as doctors; qualified properly just like all the rest of us, and then felt some kind of tug at their proverbial coat-tails, an unconscious urge maybe to give assistance to those afflicted with some mental ailment.

or 'After all, a psychiatrist is only a man or a woman – at the end of the day, that is.' And, more enigmatically, kicking and screaming out of its context: I turned to my wife and said: 'For burglar alarms, read chastity belts'. What about

'he informed me that I was 'angry, anal, and narcissistic'! The reply that I would have liked to give him would have been: "I bet you say that to all the boys!".'

or the *cri de coeur* 'I learnt much from her, mainly the ability to recognize the type, should she ever recur again in my practice.' Not to mention the charming, if irrelevant:

I am reminded of the very attractive young woman who had followed me through a series of first aid lectures. After one of these talks, she came up to me with the news that only the previous day she had seen a really dreadful accident. 'You'd have been proud of me', she said – as she told of the victim lying in a pool of blood, 'and I knew just what to do. . . .'
I nodded approvingly.
'. . . . I put my head between my knees to stop myself fainting!'

My Life Among the Monoamines

A nd how, many of you will want to know, does a chemical pathologist at a maternity hospital come to be mixing with the neuropsychiatrists? Monoamines – 5-hydroxytryptamine, catecholamines and all that jazz – form the connecting threads, down in the uterus, up in the brain and out to the Caribbean; but my love affair with the field goes deeper. In fact, I remember the exact moment when it first sparked. As a medical student in the late 1940s, the total psychiatric teaching consisted of two afternoons at the local bin (it was enough – they got it all in). At the first session, I was given a patient to clerk who had been a Lecturer in Physics. I even remember his name – John Thomas, although all the nurses called him Willie – I couldn't think why. He was a gangling, eunuchoid-looking fellow, with a strange, high-pitched quacking voice, like a cross between C.E.M. Joad (anybody remember him?) and Donald Duck.

I said, 'Has you voice always been like that?'. 'Only since the helium', he replied. He claimed that it all started when his hydrocoele was tapped and the fluid was replaced by helium. After this operation, he told me, he drifted straight up and hung upside-down from the ceiling for three days. I was rather inclined to disbelieve him. I thought he was boasting – but then I saw a picture in Bailey & Love, the surgical text book we all used to use, of a man with elephantiasis carrying his rather substantial scrotum in a wheelbarrow, so I kept an open mind.

MERTON SANDLER
London

2 Schizophrenia

F rom that first seminal day as a student to this, schizophrenia, with its protean manifestations, has never ceased to fascinate me. Take the recent case of 'Musical hallucinations' described by I. McLoughlin (British Journal of Psychiatry, 156, (1990), 452):

She continued, however, to complain of an insistent hallucinatory voice emanating from her vagina — in the form of songs being repeated over and over again, the main ones being 'The Old Rugged Cross', 'Jerusalem', and 'The Hallelujah Chorus'. . . . . . The patient was often noted to sing along with the voices; at other times they appeared to irritate her.

Of course, these days biological psychiatry rules OK and the latest, state-of-the-art model of schizophrenia is provided by certain mutant strains of slime mould. A psychiatrist from San Diego, Umberto Cohen, is the world's top expert. He is passionately interested in his subject — he says if you mix them in an omelette, they taste just like mushrooms. He came over last summer. I said to my wife, 'I'm just going to London Airport to meet Umberto Cohen'. She said 'I suppose he's flying in by El Alitalia.'

A Mars A Day

T he noun, 'nerve', can be used in pseudomedical terminology in many ways, often paradoxical. When someone remains cool in the face of considerable adversity we say that he has 'nerves of steel', yet if he does not remain calm under such circumstances we say that he is 'nervous' or 'nervy'. If a person shows gross effrontery we say that has 'nerve', and yet, if we say that he is suffering from his 'nerves' we mean something considerably different. I am reminded of something Edmund Burke once said: 'He that wrestles with us strengthens our nerves, and sharpens our skill. Our antagonist is our helper.'

Looking back on my dealings with Ron's family over the years I see that all connotations of the word 'nerve' are applicable. Ron and his wife had been patients of our long-established practice from birth and their children, and their children, were also registered with us. This would seem to be the epitome of family medicine at its best (i.e. RCGP approved!) but, unfortunately, there were drawbacks which flawed the seemingly happy picture.

Ron, when I first met him, was in his early fifties. He was tall and thin with greying hair and was almost totally edentulous. He appeared to have boundless energy as he could be seen striding around the housing estate where he lived and always walked to the surgery, three miles away, for his consultations, spurning the comfort of the buses that plied frequently into the City Centre. He originally worked as a labourer in one of the local factories, which produced sausages for the nation, but had eventually drifted into unemployment, even before that unhappy state of affairs became popular. He was also, unfortunately, schizophrenic but his disease had been quiescent for several years.

His wife was small and dumpy and always had a down-trodden look. She was the main breadwinner, with a job as a cleaner at the local junior school in the evenings and a similar job in an accountant's office in the early mornings. She had suffered from depression in her early 20s, severe enough for her to be admitted to our mental hospital and it was while she was there that she met her husband. Nowadays, her hours at home coincided with the times that her husband was on his wanderings and her cleaning duties kept her away from home while her husband was there. This was, I suspected, more than a coincidence. She had coped with her husband's illness with fortitude, especially during its more florid phases of earlier years, but had grown weary as time passed and they had drifted into a rather separate existence.

They had had two daughters in their marriage. The two girls were not alike in the slightest. The elder one lived with her two children in the same part of the town as her parents. She was a pleasant chubby girl, although not very bright. She had been impregnated by her boyfriend before marriage and, after they had legalized their relationship, they had had a second child. Unfortunately, it was inevitable that the marriage would not last and she evenutally broke up with her husband who drank a lot and was violent. She was loving and caring, in her own way, towards her family and her parents. She worked packing meat pies for her father's erstwhile employers.

The other daughter had risen in the world; she was bright at junior school and had won (in pre-comprehensive days) a scholarship to the local Girls' High School; where she had gained 5 'O' level passes and had become a secretary. While thus employed she had met her husband, a lawyer's managing clerk (I think they are known as 'legal executives' in these euphemistic days; after all am I not a 'physician in primary medical care' instead of 'family doctor?'). They lived on the other, considerably more exclusive, side of town in a new 'executive' style house (meaning jerry-built, small and almost touching next door!). She seemed slightly ashamed of her background; her children were being educated in a private junior school. She visited her parents – sometimes. She did not need to work, and she was a member of various 'select' charitable committees.

My first meeting with the family occurred shortly after I became a partner in the practice. Ron was behaving strangely and his wife was worried about his mental state. It was a miserable, dark, wet night and I did not then have an instinctive knowledge of the geography of our practice area. Also, unfortunately, the City Fathers in the 1930s, when the estate where Ron and his family lived was built, had approved house designs in which the 'front' door of the house was, in fact, on the side; and the paint scheme was dark blue front doors with black numbers, making recognition wellnigh impossible.

Because of these factors I took almost three quarters of an hour to find the house. To my horror, there were two police cars, complete with blue flashing lights, outside the front gate. Sir W. S. Gilbert thought that 'the policeman's lot is not a happy one', and, certainly, the two young constables were looking decidedly uncomfortable and wet as they waited outside the house.

Ron's wife let me in. We thought you weren't coming; that's why we called the police', she explained, showing me into the living room. 'You see,' she continued, 'he's getting radio messages from Mars!'

This symptom was slightly disconcerting, and several years as a student and then as a resident had not acquainted me with such complaints. I hesitated, wondering what I should do next. Should I call one of my experienced partners to ask their advice? On second thoughts I decided not as it might give them cause for concern about the competence of their new partner. Should I return to the surgery to look up his symptoms in my old (and that was a true description) text-book of psychiatry. However, that course of action would give Ron's wife doubts about clinical acumen. Suddenly I realized that my next step was obvious; I would have to see the patient!

He was dressed in a pair of stained trousers, accompanied by a string vest and surrounded by a mountainous pile of cigarette ends and ash. He was sitting by the hearth staring at the fireplace. I tried to initiate a conversation with him, but was impatiently quietened and told that I was interrupting his message. After a few moments he turned to me quizzically. I explained the nature of my presence and eventually I managed to elicit from him the interplanetary advice that he was receiving down the chimney. Apparently the occupants of Mars were advising him of the impending 'Second Coming'.

I soon realized that his thought processes were somewhat abnormal and that, perhaps, emergency psychiatric admission was the most appropriate course of action. I was able to contact the Mental Welfare Officer on call (this was in the distant past, you must realize) who turned up fairly promptly. He knew Ron from previous encounters and after the necessary preliminaries, he ushered Ron into the ambulance that I had ordered at the same time that I had arranged his hospital bed. I was very impressed with the cool efficiency of the experienced MWO. He was a grizzled Lancastrian who had been doing the job for years and he demonstrated an unhurried calm during his dealing with his patients.

Before the 1959 Mental Health Act, one of my partners was called out to a patient who, too, was receiving messages from God. In those days an emergency compulsory admission necessitated the signature of a magistrate, and one was duly called to officiate. To my partner's surprise he spent 40 minutes talking to the patient, before turning to my partner and asking how he knew that the patient was not receiving divine messages!

'I wondered', my partner mused later, 'which was the madder of the two of them!'

Ron was in hospital for some months before being discharged, well controlled on both oral and depot parenteral phenothiazine preparations, and apart from regular visits to the surgery for his prescriptions, injections and certificates, he rarely bothered us.

We should have realized that something was wrong when his surgery attendances became increasingly rare until they stopped altogether but, because we were used to him (and familiarity, after all, breeds contempt), we tended not to notice that he was failing to attend for his medication.

For about three years, he remained reasonably well without treatment, but this state of affairs was, alas, the calm before a very violent storm. One night when I was on call for emergencies, the crisis arrived. (I feel that all such occurrences take place on my days on duty, and my wife thinks I am the unluckiest doctor in the practice. So unfortunately, think all the practice wives about their husbands!). At around 11.30 p.m., when I was wondering whether it was safe to contemplate going to bed, I received a call from Ron's very distraught elder daughter. For a few weeks, he had been hearing voices again and, tonight, he had been ordered to kill his long-suffering wife. Initially he had tried to stab her with a kitchen knife and then, when he had failed in that attempt, he had half-strangled her. She had, fortunately, managed to escape and had sought asylum at her daughter's house. Ron, in the meantime, had stayed at home and with his wife gone, had calmed down, although he kept replying to 'the voices'.

On this occasion, when I arrived there were no police cars and, with no lack of trepidation, I entered the house. Ron was sitting very much as he had been on my previous attempt at crisis intervention.

'It's her', he said to my enquiry about his health. 'They say that she's been trying to kill me and they said that I'd better protect myself by getting her first.' I asked who 'they' were. He pointed at the fireplace and said, 'them Martians; they talk to me a lot as I'm their messenger here.'

After more conversation along these lines, it became increasingly obvious that emergency admission was again appropriate. I went to tell his family about my plan of action. His wife and elder daughter were profuse in their thanks. His younger daughter, who had by now arrived in her (as opposed to her husband's) car was less thankful.

'It's all your fault,' she said. 'If he had killed my mother, we would have got my husband's firm to sue you. People like him should be locked away permanently. They're not fit to be in decent society.'

I deflected her anger in my best Balint manner and went to 'phone the duty social worker. My call was dealt with by the disembodied voice of an answering machine; it asked me to 'phone another number in the next largest town in the County, some 90 miles to the south west. Wearily, I did just that and was answered by a person who left me in no doubt that he thought that it was an inappropriate time to contact him, and even after I explained the circumstances to him, he did not seem mollified.

'Give me your telephone number and I'll contact the social worker on call for your area. If she is in, she'll ring you,' he said.

After what seemed to be an eternity, but which was, in fact, only 40 minutes, the duty social worker 'phoned. I explained the circumstances to her, thinking that she would readily agree with my assessment, but I was disappointed.

'Is an emergency admission appropriate?' she asked. 'Yes,' I replied, pointing out that Ron had left me in no doubt that the voices were still instructing him to attack his wife.

'Are you sure it won't wait until the morning?' she persevered.

At this point I nearly got cross, but tiredness overcame my irritation, and I disagreed with her question.

'All right,' she said, obviously dissatisfied with my diagnostic and management acumen, 'I will come up and sort this mess out for you.'

I asked her how long she would be and, to my horror, found out that she was in a market town about 20 miles away. When she arrived a further three quarters of an hour later she was still obviously cross. ('I'd only been in bed for 2 hours!' I hadn't been to bed at all!). However, she did make the necessary arrangements and Ron was moved with no great difficulty back to the local mental hospital.

When he was discharged, some six months later, we were determined to learn from our experiences and we arranged for our Community Psychiatric Nurse to give Ron his depot phenothiazine preparation. He still receives these, albeit in smaller doses nowadays, and lives an uneventful and apparently contented existence with his wife. I saw them from time to time and looked after their elder daughter when, after marrying a more congenial husband than her previous model, she became pregnant. I felt that I was very much the 'family' doctor as far as she was concerned.

Her younger sister, in the meantime, had moved out of town into a new estate in what had been a small and charming village, but which was now blighted by new housing. Her new house was 'senior executive' style (i.e., as nasty as her previous one – but more expensive) and she was now president of one of her charitable committees and her photograph regularly appeared in the local paper receiving cheques and donations. I saw little of her as she tended to see one of my partners.

Two years ago, it fell to my lot to be the unfortunate partner on duty on Christmas Day. The morning was quiet and I saw three people at home (one of whom entered into the spirit of the occasion and offered me a drink saying, 'You won't be drinking on duty, will you, doctor?').

I was just sitting down to my Christmas Lunch (turkey and all the trimmings – but absolutely no alcoholic refreshment: I once did attend a patient after having a small glass of sherry. As I looked down her throat she exclaimed, 'Good grief, you smell like a brewery!') when I was disturbed by the telephone. It was Ron's younger daughter, imperiously demanding my immediate attendance on one of her children who was, she said, obviously unwell. She couldn't give any further details and it wouldn't wait until I had finished my Christmas Pudding.

With a heavy heart I drove the 5 miles to her house wondering, somewhat apprehensively, what pathology was of sufficient urgency and such vague symptomatology to need me with such haste. The narrow roads of the village were cluttered with more parked cars than usual, an indication that other families were also performing the annual ritual of entertaining their relations.

I found their house and walked up the drive; although they were expecting me they did not appear to be peering anxiously through the front windows. I rang the bell, and then rang it again after it remained unanswered. She eventually opened the door and showed me into the dining room where her husband and two children, obviously very far from unwell, were sitting at the table which was laden with food.

She pointed at me and said, to her younger child, 'See. I told you I would get the doctor to you if you didn't eat your sprouts!'

JOHN HAWORTH
Carlisle

Delusions

I learnt fairly early on in my career that there was no point in arguing with a delusion. A young patient of mine firmly believed that the Masons were entering his room at night and hypnotizing him in order to control his thoughts during the day and would not entertain any other explanation. One afternoon, he asked me if I would tell him, honestly, what I thought was wrong with him. Sensing that he might be gaining some insight, I spent a long time trying to explain that, although his experiences seemed very genuine to him, they were occurring in his mind and not in the real world. 'Are you convinced?' I asked, and he shook his head ruefully. Suddenly I had what I thought was a brilliant idea. 'All right,' I said, 'what if I told you that I had another patient who believed exactly the same things were happening to him but that it was the South African Police rather than the

Masons?' (this was not entirely true, but a bit of psychiatric licence). At this, his eyes lit up, 'I'd believe him,' he declared triumphantly', because its probably the Masons disguised as South African Police.'

ALISON JENAWAY
Cambridge

Who's Normal Anyway?

There's an old Yorkshire saying that 'everyone in this world is mad except thee and me, and I'm not so sure about thee!' It can be very difficult to diagnose certain forms of psychiatric illness, schizophrenia for example. It is not even recognized as a condition in America I understand. I will always remember my old Professor of Psychiatry saying that 'if you are ever in a consultation with a patient and start wondering whether you or the patient is mad, then you are dealing with a schizophrenic.' But he went on to say 'that is, if you are absolutely sure you are not schizophrenic!'

Our practice gave the anaesthetics for the weekly ECT sessions at the local psychiatric hospital, which was literally just down the road. One of our patients, a longstanding schizophrenic, was in again, following another of his not infrequent episodes of 'hearing other people's thoughts'. We considered him harmless, but passers-by in the street did not take it kindly when he grabbed them by the arm and told them he knew what they were thinking. His main problem was failure to take medication at home, not uncommon but fairly soon sorted out in hospital.

Usually I heard on the grapevine when he had been admitted, but this was the first time I had been asked to see any of the staff at the hospital about his problem. I wondered what had happened to cause this meeting. As I entered the superintendent's room I saw that it must be important. Not only were the ward sister and consultant psychiatrist there, but also the psychiatric social worker and hospital superintendent. Had he turned violent? – had he tried to take an overdose? – all sorts of possibilities rushed through my mind.

After the normal welcomes, the consultant psychiatrist broached the problem. Our patient was a very intelligent man, in fact he had a PhD in Biochemistry. He probably knew as much about the written word on schizophrenia as any psychiatrist, because he was interested in his condition and assiduously read up about it in his periods of normality. He was also very well read on Extra Sensory Perception (ESP). Not only was he well read, he was in contact with many of the experts in this field. Indeed, he was in frequent communication with a Professor who held a chair in Paranormal Influences, for goodness sake, at some unmemorable American University. Our patient and this Professor, apparently, had been undertaking 'research' into ESP by trying to pass their thoughts across the Atlantic Ocean.

The problem was, this 'research' had gone so well that the American Professor wanted to publish. Not only publish, but in an eminent journal. 'So what was the problem?' I asked the meeting. Our patient was to be a co-author and the hospital was to be his designated place of work. Suddenly it clicked. The American Professor thought that his co-worker into this extra-sensory research project was a psychiatrist at the hospital and had no idea he was a patient. 'Oh my goodness,' I thought, 'how splendid.' The hospital superintendent saw my expanding smile and quickly interrupted it by saying 'under no circumstances can we allow him to use this hospital's name and address. We will be the laughing stock of the whole area, not to say the whole country if the papers get to hear of it.' I thought it might provide a very good story for *The News of the World* or some other such newspaper. But I agreed in the end of course and it turned out that I was the chosen one to pass on the news. He could use his home address and there would be no communication by the hospital with the American professor, but no mention or use at all of the hospital as his place of work or address.

I saw him in an ante-room. As soon as he walked in he looked at me and said 'I know what you are thinking.' And he did!

B. T. MARSH
Chalfont St Peter

Restraining Oneself

Although 'voices' are sometimes comforting, most auditory hallucinations seem to be distressing. They may be annoying, worrying or frightening. It certainly does not give patients a sense of empathy and understanding if their psychiatrists burst into laughter when told about such impositions on their patient's sensoria.

Usually I have no trouble holding back my mirth. Indeed, I commonly feel empathically upset or angry about the voices. The content may be absurd, and I wonder what process within the brain could cause such ideas to erupt into consciousness without an external stimulus. Just occasionally, in reaction to an apparently undistressed patient's account, I will feel amused and I will know I must not laugh – which makes it all the harder to stop the corners of my mouth rebelling, and all the other actions which contribute to the laughter process from taking place. I do try, I really do! And if resistance seems impossible I take out my handkerchief with a flourish (scattering previously expressed germs all over my patient, no doubt) and blow loudly. No doubt you do the same.

I failed with Mrs B. She was a pleasant, bright, but not very intelligent lady in her sixties. I'd seen her before and diagnosed paraphrenia. Her personality was well preserved. On one of her visits to me she was quite angry. 'They've been at me again,' she complained. 'Down Oxford Street. They were following me – but every time I turned round, they hid. And do you know what they said? ''Bumberclod'',' she told me indignantly. '''Bumberclod'' and ''Pots and pans'''.

I took out my handkerchief.

She looked at me quizzically and then went on 'They kept on doing it all down the street. And then, do you know what they said?' She sounded really offended, so I strained to think what it might be. '''Tupperware!''' she said.

I blew my nose.

JOHN SNOWDON
Australia

Trouble with the Neighbours

Maisie Finch had always been one of life's worriers. As she sat in my waiting room that morning she looked older than her 49 years. Caring for her mother had not helped. She had nursed the irascible old lady at home for over five years. Last summer a second stroke had provided a merciful release for both parties. However, now that nine months had passed, I had hoped to see less of Maisie. She had coped quite well with her bereavement, and now that spring was in the air, I was rather disappointed to see her back once again. As she came in and sat down, she had about her that same anxiety that had always accompanied her numerous consultations about old Mrs Finch. My disappointment turned to concern as she told me why she had come to see me.

'Oh, you know me, Doctor, I'm fine. Strong as an ox. Had to be, didn't I, to look after Mum all that time. No, it's Mr Bradshaw I'm worried about.'

My puzzlement must have shown. Some of my patients are always surprised that, even after four years in Kelton, I have still not memorized the names, faces, ailments and addresses of every one of the town's inhabitants.

'You know, him in number 33. My next door neighbour.'

'Oh.' Where was all this leading? I had a nasty suspicion that it was going to be a long consultation, my pen doodled slowly across the blotter.

'He's been acting very strange lately, Doctor. The radio I could put up with, but I thought I'd better let you know about the bore-holes and the poison gas.'

She paused, which was nice of her, because it gave me plenty of time to stop counting the leaves on my rubber plant, look at Miss Finch, realize that she was, as ever, deadly serious, and then think of something to say. 'Err, this Mr Bradshaw, his radio. He plays it very loudly does he? Music at all hours, that sort of thing?' 'Well, yes and no. It is usually in the middle of the night, but it's not music, it's voices.' 'Voices? What do these voices say Maisie?' 'Well. Often I'm not sure, it's not too clear. But I always feel as if they're talking to me. Telling me to do things. Strange things.'

I had stopped doodling now, my pen was poised to record Maisie's account. This was getting more and more interesting.

'Could you give me an example?' 'Well, last night, for instance. I was lying in bed and this voice said "You must go to the station", just like it was right inside my head. They often tell me to go places, these voices.'

This was sounding less like a troublesome neighbour and more like acute schizophrenia every second. I probed on gently. 'You haven't been out much, have you, since your mum died? Don't you feel that you might not like to, you know, spread your wings a bit now? It must be a bit depressing for you, sitting around at home all day. . .' 'Oh no, Doctor, I don't mind. And anyway, I really feel that I have to keep an eye on that Mr Bradshaw, especially since the bore-holes.' 'Ah, yes, these bore-holes. Perhaps you'd better tell me about them.'

Underneath 'thought insertion and passivity' I wrote 'paranoid delusions' whilst Maisie went on to relate how her neighbour was, very quietly, drilling small holes through their party wall in order to spy on her. She told me how the voices had become louder since the spy-holes had appeared, and how she felt that she could cope with that but, now that Mr Bradshaw was pumping poison gas through to her bedroom, she felt that she really ought to come and see me.

I tried to persuade Maisie to accept a prescription for 'something to help her sleep', but she politely declined my offer. Sleep was not a problem and, now that she had let me know about poor Mr Bradshaw, she would be on her way. 'Dear Mother always had such faith in you. I'm sure that you'll be able to sort this out. He used to be such a nice man too. He keeps Highland terriers, you know. Goodbye Doctor.'

I was left in a quandary. The poor woman was plainly in need of help, but she had absolutely no insight into her plight at all. Who knew what harm might come to her, or her neighbour, if no one intervened?

The following day I 'just happened' to be passing Miss Finch's neat Victorian semi-detached home. Gingerly, I rang the polished brass door bell. For a long time nothing happened. I scanned the outside of the house. There appeared to be no sign of life behind the carefully arranged lace curtains. Still no answer, and I glanced across at the neighbouring house. Sadly, I noted that, far from being inhabited by a wall-drilling poisoner, Number 33, Harlowe Crescent seemed to have stood empty for some time. Its grimy windows and leaf-strewn porch contrasted strongly with the prim cleanliness of my patient's house.

I thought that I heard a shuffle in the hallway so, in time-honoured family doctor style, I bent down to squint through the letter box. 'Miss Finch,' I called 'are you there? It's the doctor.'

A touselled mop of hair poked out from one of the doorways. I made further reassuring noises and eventually persuaded a very suspicious Maisie to open the door. My instincts had been right, the poor woman had obviously deteriorated in the space of a single day. Gently I asked if she had had any further trouble. She shot fearful glances around the hallway as she told me how the poison gas smell was getting worse, and the voices louder still. Last night they had been telling her to drive to Buckley Reservoir and jump in. 'But Doctor,' she tailed off sadly, 'Buckley's 25 miles away, and I don't even have a car.'

Whatever faint hope I had of calming her paranoia was rapidly fading, but I asked her to show me her bedroom anyway. Perhaps I could demonstrate to her that the walls were solid and intact. She seemed almost pathetically grateful for the suggestion and scurried up the gloomy staircase before me like a little grey mouse.

She had continued to sleep in the back bedroom since her mother's death. As I stood on the threshold I found that, despite myself, I sniffed the air speculatively. Nothing but the smell of air-freshener pervaded the room. The net curtains billowed in the breeze. Maisie followed my glance. 'I have to have the window open all night, or I'd surely have been overcome by now Doctor.'

I turned to the wall that she claimed was peppered with bore-holes. A huge mahogany wardrobe filled most of the space between the corner fireplace and the door. It looked massively immovable, especially by someone of Maisie's stature. 'Ah, you see what I've had to do to stop

Mr Bradshaw. I thought that mother's wardrobe would be the answer, but it didn't work. Look!'

Suddenly my patient collapsed on the carpet. I stepped forward, full of concern. Then I realized that she was pointing at something underneath the wardrobe. A quick scan of the skirting board with the aid of my medical torch revealed nothing more sinister than a rather large mouse hole. I tried to explain this to Maisie, but for the first time she looked at me with ice in her eyes.

'Doctor.' She drew herself up to her full height (five-foot-two in her stockinged feet according to our notes) 'Do I look like the sort of woman that would suffer rodents in my house?' I had to admit that she did not. I left, suitably chastened, and promised to call again the next day to do something about her troublesome neighbour. Back in the car I added 'suicidal thoughts' to her list of symptoms.

As soon as I was back at the surgery I tried to contact our local psychiatrist to arrange an urgent domiciliary visit for the following day. It was the usual story after my call was put

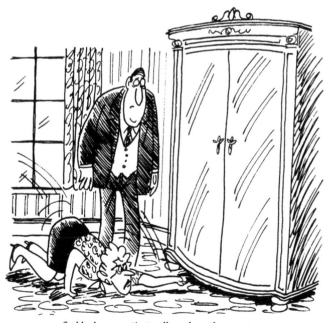

Suddenly my patient collapsed on the carpet.

through to his office in St Cecilia's. No, Dr Epstein was not
in the hospital at present. No, his secretary could not tell me
when he would be back. This was because his secretary was
off sick and the girl I was talking to had only started that day.
Yes, she supposed that she could arrange for Dr Epstein to
meet me at Miss Finch's house the next afternoon, but it
really was difficult to say definitely. She thought he would be
free at two but the diary was really in a shocking state. All
right, I would be 'pencilled in', but she would have to ring
me back if there was any problem. It was almost a relief to
start afternoon surgery.

To my suprise, the only call of the afternoon came, not from
St Cecilia's but from Maisie herself. Our receptionist had
been unable to cope with her and so had patched her through
to me in between Wayne Carter's verrucae and Mr Simpson's
diabetes check.

She seemed remarkably calm as she told me how the voices
in her head had multiplied, and begun shouting and swear-
ing at her. The banging on the walls had been terrible too. But
it was all right now, it had all stopped. No, she did not think
that I need bother to see her again today, but she had thought
that I would like to know.

I gave my partner a brief résumé of the day's events as I
went off duty that evening, and Maisie's notes joined the
select box full of those 'on the boil' patients likely to require
an out-of-hours visit. I hoped not, but one never knew.

As I drove home I slowly relaxed. At last I could stop
worrying about my patients' incipient psychoses and
concentrate on less stressful matters. That night I was
meeting Fred Martin, from the Northolt Street practice, for
our weekly game of squash.

A couple of hours later we were both resting our aching
limbs in The Crooked Billet, restoring our fluid and
electrolyte balance with a couple of pints of 'Old Peculiar'.
We had both joined partnerships in Kelton at around the
same time and our regular matches were a good excuse for
picking over together the mutual grievances of a doctor's lot.

The conversation turned to the general lousiness of the
local hospitals' switch-boards and ill-concealed animosity of
most consultants' secretaries. I related my experience at the
hands of Dr Epstein's temp. Fred was mildly surprised. He

told me that Doreen, Epstein's usual girl, was a model of efficiency. He then told me about Billy, a recently retired butcher. Dr Epstein had been really helpful with this sad case of Fred's, but, despite their best efforts, they had had to admit him forcibly for treatment that very afternoon. 'Classic case of schizophrenia. Normally a lovely chap, but since he retired, stranger and stranger. Single you see. I reckon it's often the loneliness that tips them over the edge.' I nodded in silent agreement. How right he was. 'Only had his pets, but that's not the same is it? He needed someone to talk to, but he was too shy. Everything went to rack and ruin. Started hearing voices, reckoned his neighbours were out to get him. As for his house. Well, it was a mess on the outside, but the bedroom; I nearly threw up.' 'We were round there today, old Epstein and I. It needed both of us and the ambulance men to get him out. Of course, the social worker wasn't keen to section him, but when we showed him that room he soon changed his mind.' 'A bit smelly was it?' Funny how every case was different, I recalled Miss Finch's spotless boudoir.

'It was the dogs.' 'Dogs?' Some where deep in my off-duty psyche alarm bells were starting to ring. 'Yes, a couple of terriers I think. He'd locked the poor creatures in there with him. I think that he'd probably killed them. It was difficult to tell, they'd been dead a long time.' Frank pinched his nose demonstratively. 'Old Billy had built up this sort of shelter around them, had this old radio set, "to be ready for the invaders" he reckoned. Telescope at the window. He'd even started digging into the wall, drilling into the plaster with an old screwdriver. Sends shivers down my spine even now, thinking about the weeks he must have spent up there. All alone with those two dead mutts and that valve radio tuned to the local taxi frequency. Dig, dig, dig all night. No wonder his neighbour called me in. Nice woman, one of your patients I think, can't quite recall her name at the moment. Here, are you all right? Anyone would think that you'd seen a ghost!'

Miss Finch did not call out my partner that night. In the morning I rang St. Cecilia's to cancel Dr Epstein's visit. The temp. was still there; she was not impressed. 'Dr Epstein told me he'd already admitted the patient from Harlowe Crescent, but I told him you said it was urgent. He reckoned that I'd

got things mixed up, and now you say you don't want him
to go anyway! I wish you'd make your mind up! Sometimes
it's hard to know who's mad and who isn't 'round here.'

I was about to voice a suitably cutting rejoinder, but then
I thought better of it. After all, she was absolutely right.

GERAINT JONES
Leiston

First Psychiatric Patient

M y first psychiatric patient was nearly my last.
When I walked into the last terrace house at the
bottom of Derman Road, past the note on the door inviting
me to come straight in, John was clearly visible through the
open door leading into the back room. He was pinning his
father to the wall, with a large Sabatier knife held menacingly
against his throat.

My first reaction was to run, rationalizing my cowardice
with the 'sensible' decision to get further help, but when the
terrified father said, 'Thank heavens you've come doctor,
John has great faith in you,' I set my bag down and inwardly
cursed the cold snap of 1958.

It was during the cold months of January and February of
that year that I was supposed to learn about mental disorder
at a beautiful country hospital, set amidst rolling hills. In
those days psychiatry was viewed with great suspicion by the
other consultants, and especially the surgeons, whose
simplistic view of life was that 'if it hurt, cut it out'. Somehow
the insidious propaganda of the surgeons must have
conditioned our attitudes, so that even the keenest students
began to regard this part of our course as some light relief
from the rigours of the pre-final months.

Thus a great deal of the time that should have been spent
on schizophrenia was, instead, spent on toboggans and skis,
going down the snow-covered slopes surrounding the
hospital.

Which didn't help much when John turned his attention to me, and while he didn't actually pin me to the wall, he stood with the knife held threateningly in the underarm position, favoured by those who know that an overarm attack is more easily countered.

I did the only thing I could, I talked; and I kept talking. During the next 30 minutes' discourse on God, the weather and Derby County, the tension gradually eased, and I began to think that perhaps I was lucky to have missed a great deal of the formal instruction in psychiatry. Maybe common sense and instinct were best after all.

My complacency was suddenly shattered by the arrival of the police, fetched by a breathless mother, who had only paused long enough on her way out to pin that innocuous note on the door, the one inviting me blandly to disaster.

The long arm of the law was all for reaching rapidly towards the offender and ending the situation in a quick scuffle, but as I was nearest the knife I dissuaded them, pretending superior medical knowledge. This was, after all, my first job as a trainee G.P. and I didn't want to end what I thought would be a long and industrious career, in a pool of blood under a Trechikoff print and a line of alabaster ducks.

After a further hour's tense small talk, I eventually persuaded John to come with me in my Green A.40 to the nearby psychiatric hospital, where proper treatment and kind attention were available. As we were leaving I just managed to whisper to John's father that I would welcome the help of a couple of strong porters when we got there, just in case.

We moved off, thankfully leaving the knife behind, and as we got nearer the hospital my spirits gradually rose, as I looked forward to imminent release and a much-needed pint in the local hostelry.

On our arrival, I persuaded John to get out of the car, and as we walked towards the main door, two burly figures in navy blue moved smartly down the steps and towards us. Of the sudden flurry of events which followed my memory is fortunately hazy. But I do remember being seized, one strong grip on each arm, and being rushed up the steps protesting desperately that I was the doctor, while John stood meekly at the bottom, looking as harmful as a spring lamb and even less interested.

Later that night I looked long and hard at the face staring back at me from the mirror, and wondered what vital nugget of psychiatric learning I had missed during that long cold spell in 1958.

S.E. ANNESLEY
Nottingham

Jan the Schizophrenic

Jan, the schizophrenic, had gone mad again. She was unable to look after herself and her neglect had resulted in obvious vitamin deficiencies. She was anaemic and her gums were bleeding from lack of vitamin C. Her husband had seen it all before and had reluctantly called for help.

I met the newly-appointed consultant outside the house. He was smartly dressed, wearing a warm woollen overcoat. The social worker had on jeans and an anorak. We walked to the house along a cracked concrete path overgrown with weeds and under a broken-down trellis arch which was covered with the dying remnants of a rambler rose.

The consultant walked with a spring in his step, certificates under his arm, towards the front door. He promptly trod in the droppings of the neighbouring cat who found the overgrown garden an irresistible happy hunting ground for small birds and a repository for giving something back to nature.

We were shown by the husband into the front room which was typical of the council houses built in the 1930s. Jan was manically ironing clothes in front of the fire. She was dirty, unkempt and looked as if she had lost weight. Her eye caught the consultant's. As if to calm her down, he sat in the armchair by the fireplace. Its springs had long since died of fatigue. His knees ended up higher than his head as he descended into the depths of the unsupported upholstery. He struggled on its sides using his elbows to relieve his dignity and from then on sat on a still-preserved arm.

Jan remained silent but eyed him steadily. Then came the usual questions about hearing voices, were people looking at her and talking about her, and whether she was doing the housework and shopping. At first she answered with a yes or no, looking increasingly perplexed as the interview progressed. Gradually her resentment showed through and finally she exploded in a mixture of her native Polish and unflattering Anglo-Saxon.

The husband remained impassive. The social worker looked intense and caring. After all, he had to look after the patient's rights. The previous consultant, who had just retired, was a reassuring grey-haired old man who knew all about eye contact. This one had provoked her by the way he carried himself and addressed her. She made a dash for the door and was through it running towards the fields and neighbouring disused cement quarries.

The village had been making cement for 200 years. It was surrounded by man-made lakes which had resulted from the quarrying. There were also scrub, woods, a nature reserve and the remains of a cement works which had been dynamited by the army 20 years ago. It was the perfect place for hiding out. It was the end of December and the middle of a cold spell. The consultant and social worker decided that it was in the best interests of the patient that she should be taken to a place of safety as soon as possible and not left hiding out in the countryside. The police were summoned. A search should be started as soon as possible. Unfortunately, most of them were off-duty on their Christmas break. The local sergeant arrived and took charge of the situation.

It just so happened that a local derby football match was taking place on the village playing field. It was being watched by most of the village people who were also taking an extended break during Christmas and the new year. The police decided to ask for volunteers.

Most were merry from the festivities. They gradually gathered around the police for instructions. Most wore anoraks and jeans. One parent in a light-blue track suit was showing off ball control to his son and slipped on the mud. He now had a large brown patch on his seat. His son was repeatedly wiping a large viscous ball of snot from his nose

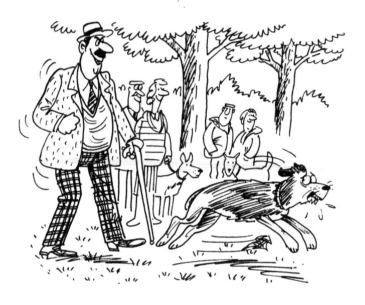

It bit his leg and then ran away yelping as it found it artificial.

on to his sleeve. Several volunteers repeatedly drank from hip flasks.

There were dogs everywhere. A Rottweiler with a look of malice on its face took a dislike to a man with a limp. It bit his leg and then ran away yelping as it found it artificial. The man grinned at its owner. A fight had developed between a Jack Russell and an Alsatian. 'Pity the poor Alsatian' somebody muttered. The little dog lunged between the Alsatian's hind legs and grabbed his testicles, then hung on for all his life was worth. When he finally let go the Alsatian retired to lick his wounds. A pure-bred Labrador was mounted by a lop-eared sheep-dog with a greyhound's tail much to their owners' embarrassment. There were dogs chasing rabbit scent, dogs scratching holes and dogs defaecating. They seemed to anticipate a good afternoon's fun. As it turned out, for us humans like poor Jan, it became demented.

We walked along the lane from the playing field towards the site of the quarries and old cement works. A mini drove past full of youngsters, its windows steamed up so it was doubtful whether it could see where it was going. It pulled over on to the verge and wound down its window to find out what was happening. It had parked on a large muddy hump. When it set off its wheels rotated without effect, like a small child's legs when it is picked up by a reprimanding adult. With a whoop of joy several searchers rushed forwards to push it off. As the mini tipped forwards allowing its wheels to bite, they were spattered with mud; faces, anoraks, jeans and all. Shrieks of encouragement from the occupants blended with abuse from the pushers.

Word had got around about the search. The ghouls had already started to arrive to watch. One couple arrived in a spotless new car. Meanwhile the Alsatian had regained its dignity and was out for revenge. The Jack Russell headed for the ghouls' car and leapt on to the bonnet and then the roof. The Alsatian was not so agile, and standing on its hind legs pawed its way all round the car. The side of the car was covered with large muddy paw marks, the roof and bonnet smaller ones. It was psychedelic in a dirty sort of way. The occupants were obviously yelling from inside the car. We could see their mouths moving but their voices were drowned by the barking. Eventually the Jack Russell slipped off the roof and the chase continued up the lane.

The search began near several lagoons left from the limestone excavations. Nearby piles of discarded blue lias clay had been fenced off at one time but someone had stolen the barbed wire. The piles of clay were very slippery in the wet. Even a 'Danger' sign was leaning drunkenly towards the bottom of their slopes. It had been helped on its way by numerous air rifle pellets.

We lined up at the edge of the scrub ten yards apart. The police sergeant stood at the end, reviewing the line and shouting instructions. So intent on his new found task was he that he stepped sideways into a partially-hidden ditch, which had a foot or so of water in the bottom. There were hoots of derision from those of the villagers who had previously crossed him.

A dead elm provided a diversion for an inebriated group of searchers at the end of the line. It was already leaning and they wanted to push it over. As they arched it backwards and forwards, bits of branch, half cylinders of dead bark and woodworm dust showered down on them. There was a deep, dull thud as the last dead root broke and the tree toppled over. With it toppled its destroyers into a heap at the bottom of the hole left by the tree. Their drunken cheers accompanied the crashing of the tree as it flattened several hawthorn bushes. Some of the watchers were not so amused. It had blocked a popular public footpath.

One of the copses that we searched bordered on to a field of winter barley. As the line of searchers emerged from the trees, a man on a Japanese three-wheeler approached them at high speed from one of the field's farm gates. He was obviously upset and was shouting about his pheasants being disturbed. The searchers were not interested. They explained about Jan. He made it clear he was not interested in the behaviour of a mad woman. At this muttered lack of sympathy he took his frustration out on the three-wheeler. As he started he let out the clutch, revved up his engine, and turned to go back across the field. He hit a bump and turned over, landing face down in the soft mud. Part of the search took place in the nature reserve. It had a large notice at the edge saying 'Nature Reserve', which some joker had changed into 'Nature Reserved For Me'. As we searched across it, we came across a group of serious-looking men and women who were looking for life in the winter leaf mould. Each had a haversack and wore boots with long woollen socks. They were upset to see us and asked us to get out of the nature reserve. They quietened down as we explained what we were doing. However, some of the dogs had been excited by the raised tone of our voices. The lop-eared sheep-dog with the greyhound's tail grabbed one of their sticks and raced away through the trees. Unfortunately, it was too long to go through a gap between two saplings. The dog fell and yelped with pain as the stick was forced back into the corners of its mouth. It ran off, leaving the stick behind, with its long tail curled up between its legs.

By the late afternoon we had covered most of the several hundred acres of old workings. The searchers who were not getting tired through physical effort were being anaethetized by their hip flasks. Suddenly a shout went up. A scraggy-looking fox ran past the end of the line of searchers. This was followed in the distance by the sound of a hunting horn and, the baying of the hounds. The Warwickshire Hunt were not very far away. Shortly, all hell broke loose. The dogs, which had previously been engaged in all sorts of diverse activities, joined forces to chase it. They the hounds arrived well ahead of the huntsmen. They joined in the chase. The huntsmen sensing that a kill was imminent, speeded up. One arrived by jumping clean over a ghoul's car. Another was shouting at the searchers to call off their dogs. Yet another was brandishing his whip at the young consultant who was obviously anti-blood sports by his comments about the hunt. Meanwhile the dogs had disposed of the fox and, being in an overexcited state, started fighting with the hounds. The Rottweiler was frustrated because his owner had put a muzzle on it. All it could do was drool with anticipation of the bites it could not inflict. The Jack Russell had attached itself to one of the pack leaders. It fought shoulder to shoulder with its erstwhile enemy, the Alsatian. Their owners were shouting abuse at the huntsmen. The drunken group still covered in woodworm dust were being horsewhipped by a huntsman as they shouted in encouragement of the dog fight. They did not mind as they could not feel anything.

The police had had enough. Their efforts at saving the schizophrenic had come to nothing, except provide a good day's fun for the villagers and their dogs. It was beginning to get dark. There was a murmur of disappointment as they called it off. Even the dogs looked sad.

The police sergeant, consultant, social worker and myself walked back to Jan's house in silence. The husband had returned earlier and was just as unconcerned as when she ran off. 'No luck then, I'm not surprised. She can be pretty crafty when she wants to. Would you like a cup to tea?' In a few minutes we were cradling hot mugs of tea in our hands. All of us were lost in our thoughts, reflecting on what had happened. I replayed some of the events of the afternoon in my mind's eye. Through my daydream, the corner of the cupboard moved. I caught the husband's eye and nodded to him to look down. It moved again. He opened it and we found Jan curled up in the bottom. A mindless grin greeted us. The perfect end to a perfect day.

JOHN SHENKMANS
Rugby

3 General Psychiatry: the Rest

As I said before, I got a pretty good grounding in psychiatry as a student. Still, after forty-odd years, you get a bit rusty, so I asked this young Saudi psychiatrist working in the lab, the one who described the cheese effect following sheep's eyes, to give me a brush-up on life events in depressive illness. He said, 'Er, well, life events – you know, birth, castration, death . . .'

Apart from schizophrenia and depression, psychiatrists are also into alcohol, food, drugs and, of course, sex – into which I myself have certain insights, working as I do at a maternity hospital. ('Did you always want to be a bacteriologist?' our Dean asked the prune-faced lady candidate, at a job interview. 'I prefer to call myself a gynaecological microbiologist,' she said rather sniffily. Quick as a flash – if you'll excuse the expression – he asked, 'Does that mean you study microorgasms?')

When my children were very young, I overheard the youngest, in scandalized tones, asking the oldest, 'Did mum and dad really do that?' 'Yes,' he said gravely, 'They did'. 'How many times?' 'Four, of course. There are four of us, aren't there?'

At that time, we always had French au pair girls. I was alarmed, soon after a new one appeared, to hear the 15 year-old say to the 11 year-old 'You know that she's a tresbian.' I said to my wife, 'Do you think it right for children to come into contact with a girl like that? By the way, what's a tresbian?' 'Ask the kid,' my wife replied. I did 'It's because she says, '"Tres bien, tres bien," all the time!'

That summer, we drove down to the French Alps and stopped off at Evian les Bains. The following day, the 11 year-old girl asked out of the blue, 'Dad, what are lesbians?' I looked at my wife, she looked at me, and I embarked on a rambling explanation of how some ladies liked other ladies instead of men. The child eyed me strangely. 'By the way,' I said 'why do you ask?' 'It's just that the sign outside the town we went to yesterday said "Evian Lesbians" and I didn't know what it meant.'

Nowadays, everything is out in the open. I had a visit from a young Chinese psychiatrist working at George's. He said 'you jogger, me pederast,' just as casually as you might say 'me Tarzan, you Jane.' Well, I thought to myself, it takes all sorts. Autres temps, autres moeurs, as I'm sure I shall be saying in 1992. Each *to his own form of exercise: after all, it says in* The Sunday Times *colour supplement that sex takes up 200 calories − this is the basis of the Sandler diet. He said, 'I bicycle pederast. Every day. From Crapham to St George's Hospital.'*

Out to Lunch

'Uh huh, Uh huh. Hmmmmm. Uh huh. Yes. Uh huh. Hmmmmm. Yes I know. Uh huh.' I cradled the telephone between neck and shoulder leaving my hands free for what, at the moment, seemed more pressing and relevant than this particular telephone conversation: pouring a coffee. 'So what was it this time?' I asked as I stirred. The ennui was not concealed from my voice, nor was it meant to be. 'Turpentine? Weedkiller? Washing-up liquid?' I took a sip as the reply came; then a spray of coffee arced over my desk and splattered onto some case notes, smudging the meticulously chronicled history of Mr Wright's compulsion repeatedly to turn off dripping taps.

'Hah!' I exclaimed with disbelief. 'Hah, that's a good one!' This conveyed the fact that, as a psychiatry SHO, I had heard most things, but not all, and I was not above being mildly amused, or impressed, or both. 'Slug pellets! Great!' I vainly tried to unsmudge the notes. 'Pity she's not a slug.'

The voice at the other end of the telephone ignored my remark and continued what seemed a fairly well-rehearsed speech. Slug pellets, it seemed, were not harmful in the quantity consumed. And, that fact having been ascertained, and all other things being equal, and what with the pressure on beds and everything, well, she was no longer a medical problem. 'So,' continued the house physician, 'since she still seems a suicide risk, we'd like you to assess her. I understand she's well known to your department.'

To be well know generally implies a state of celebrity, something, perhaps, to aspire to. To be well known to a hospital department means something entirely different: it implies a disease so rare as to render the patient famous, or so mundane and repetitive as to bore the pants off the admitting team. To be well known to the psychiatric department is a downright indictment.

With a slightly unnecessary tone of desperation, he repeated,' . . . I mean, I think she is actually very well known to you.'

'Yes, she's well known to us,' I said wearily. 'We'll come and see her. Today.'

Linda Stevens. Thirty. Divorced. Occasionally mad, more often simply bad. Well known to us. Able to cope with ripples upon the pond of life only by throwing in a depth charge in the form of a self-administered poison. This would inevitably require her admission to hospital. Her attempts were never serious enough to lead to her demise. But always sufficiently novel to provoke bemused calls to a Poisons Unit to enquire if, say, a bushel load of mothballs might be harmful to anyone other than a moth. If the act of attempted suicide has a direct opposite, then we believed that Linda had attained it the day she took two hundred vitamin tablets. The bottle claimed that three a day would make you sparkle with vitality. One therefore might have expected Linda to have radiated energy like some psychotic beacon. But she looked just the same as ever.

I replaced the 'phone long enough to regain the dialling tone, then called my consultant, Dr Webb. 'It's Linda,' I said gravely. 'And this time it's slug pellets.'

Linda Stevens, I'm sorry to use you in this way. But you provided me with the funniest episode of my life. Not amusing, or wry, or witty, but funny in a joyous, sun shining, birds singing, spring in the step sort of way. The sort of funny which brings a smile to my face whenever I think of it, every time, even now, even as I write. This is how.

I was enjoying my SHO post in psychiatry. Absolute enjoyment would have been too strong a term, but the relative enjoyment, compared to the preceding torture of obstetrics and gynaecology, was boundless. And psychiatrists, though subject to their fair share of traditional interdepartment jibes, seem to inspire a curious reaction amongst other 'normal' doctors, somewhere between suspicion and awe, a reaction I thoroughly enjoyed and possibly cultivated. This stems from their calm self-confidence, bordering on smugness, an aura of wry knowledge which extends far down the psychiatric ranks, blessing even the humble SHO. It is as if psychiatrists are party to some profound, enlightening secret. Such is the effect of adequate sleep.

As I walked to my consultant's office, I nodded to the various patients who were shambling along the corridor, each manifesting some defect as an emblem of their illness: a slipper missing, a blank expression, a curious mumble. This was normal. 'Have you watered the plants yet today Simon?' I asked. Simon was one of my patients, like so many others, of indeterminate diagnosis. As part of his occupational therapy programme, he had recently been appointed plant monitor. He lifted up his palm in an odd gesture of threatening welcome and swore at me. He then asked me for a cigarette. This, too, was normal. I told him, as I did every morning, that I did not smoke and therefore could not oblige. His palm drooped and his fingers formed an unambiguous gesture. Normal. Then he shuffled off. Down the corridor, Dr Webb opened his door. He saw me and then looked beyond me. Ominously, the shuffling had stopped and a hiss of water was audible. Simon was urinating over a Yucca. This most definitely was not normal.

'Be sure you do the others too, Simon,' called Dr Webb, never one to be nonplussed. Then quietly, to me: 'I'll get him for that later.' Dr Webb invariably appeared busy and distracted, regardless of actual workload. Throwing a spanner in his day's work in the form of Linda Stevens lent some justification to his overworked frown. Lunch was beckoning and, as the canteen was adjacent to the medical wards on the other side of the hospital, he suggested seeing Linda by way of preprandial entertainment.

I agreed. One of the many pleasing aspects of psychiatry included the close liaison between consultants and junior staff. As an SHO in other specialities, it had sometimes proved necessary for me to reintroduce myself to my superiors at regular intervals. But during psychiatry, with frequent ward rounds, case conferences and out-patient clinics, I saw Dr Webb at least once a day. And he was keen to be involved in all referrals from other hospital departments. Our assessments of patients would follow a familiar pattern: we would interview the patient together, then huddle in private, American Football style, to formulate

a management plan in which I would nod sagely at his
suggestions, finally returning to the patient like a jury with
a unanimous verdict.

As we made our way to the medical wards, I prepared
myself for the words, 'Shortly before you joined us. . .' Dr
Webb like to fill all potential silences with some news or
reminiscence, and this brisk jog across the hospital grounds
was to be no exception. 'Shortly before you joined us. . .' he
began. I smiled. So much seemed to have happened shortly
before I joined the psychiatric department; it must have been
an interesting and hectic time, and I felt a trifle guilty that so
little seemed to be happening now. I wondered ruefully if my
successor would be the recipient of many 'Shortly before you
joined us' stories. And 'shortly', though grammatically
offbeam, seemed unerringly accurate as a description of my
consultant, a person of below average height, constantly
running to a tight schedule. Shortly to arrive, shortly to
leave, shortly in stature, and so on. His lack of height was
accentuated by his weight. Respect and admiration prevent
me from describing him as fat. Well-built. Stocky. Ample.
97th centile. Portly. Shortly and portly. But neither his
lack of height nor his excess of weight were his most remarkable features. Nor were his approachability, intelligence or
geniality, though he possessed these attributes in abundance.
Most memorable, in fact, was his bottom. It is difficult,
though necessary, to describe his bottom. Him being stout
and it being in proportion, it might be described accurately as
rounded. But it was much more than a shape or size. It had
a dynamic quality. It was busy. It was in more of a hurry than
the rest of his body, which was already rushing. As it bustled
here and there, it appeared to have far more pressing things
to do than act simply as a rump. So the curious trio hurried
towards the medical block. Myself, stiff-limbed and stooped
in a slightly deferential posture. Dr Webb, shortly and portly,
hurrying his ample frame determinedly along as he re-
counted his tale. And his buttocks, fighting desperately for
the lead.

'Shortly before you joined us,' he said, 'there was an
incident on one of the orthopaedic wards. A young lady was
referred to us because she had jumped off a balcony in a
suicide bid; she broke both her legs and ended up in traction.

Perhaps we were a bit blasé in our response, a little slow getting over there. . .' His pace had slowed and it was clear that the story was timed to coincide with our arrival at the medical block, which loomed ahead. 'We completely forgot that the orthopaedic ward is on the eighth floor.' A troubled look darkened his features. 'Somehow, she got herself out of traction, hobbled to the nearest window, and. . . well, you can guess the rest.' 'Hmmmmm,' I said, trying to convey shock, sympathy for the patient, and a non-judgemental attitude towards the relevant medical and psychiatric staff; quite a feat for a nondescript noise.

He opened the door for me. 'And do you know where you land if you throw yourself off the eighth floor orthopaedic ward in this hospital?' I sneaked a look at his expression to be sure that this was a rhetorical question. I shook my head. 'Well, she came crashing through the roof of casualty,' he said, following me in. His face had brightened. 'She landed smack in the middle of the minor ops. theatre. Except, by then, she wasn't a minor op. And do you know what?'

I shook my head more emphatically this time to demonstrate that my incredulity knew no bounds.

'She survived! Amazing! God knows what the casualty staff thought. Bit of an extreme way to beat the two hour wait. Still, from then on, we've always been prompt about seeing our referrals, especially those above ground level.'

Linda Stevens was on ground level. If she had her way, she told us, she would actually have been below ground level – about ten feet under, in fact. There had been the usual sub-clinical stir when we had arrived on the medical ward. The reaction of general nursing staff to psychiatrists shifts through discernible phases: disorientation, for here are assertive people without white coats acting like medical staff. Who are they? Comprehension as we introduce ourselves with an enigmatic smile. 'We are the psychiatrists.' And a final, amused confusion. So these are the shrinks, what should we do with them? A palpable thrill runs through the ward freezing, momentarily, staff and patients, fed by knowing glances, winks and notes passed surreptitiously from bed to bed: mind what you say, the psychiatrists are here! Then, our moment of paralytic glory over, we are virtually ignored. Our presence is only registered by the fact that all the staff are smirking.

Linda had a room to herself. She was chaotic. She lived a chaotic life-style with a chaotic chronic schizophrenic called John, in what can only be described as chaos. Her appearance, her hair, her make-up – all chaotic. We listened with rapt attention as she outlined her last particular acute on chronic chaotic episode. It seemed that, after a typically violent bout of arguing, she had stormed out of their flat. However, pacing the streets clad only in dressing gown and slippers, her mood had apparently changed and she had returned to the flat bearing a peacemaking present for John.

'What did you buy him?' asked Dr Webb. Linda paused, then replied, very deliberately, 'A tortoise. I bought him a tortoise.' I shifted position in my seat. Dr Webb's face betrayed no flicker of amusement. 'But Linda,' he said, 'You live on the tenth floor of a block of flats.' I have always been impressed by a psychiatrist's detailed knowledge of his patients. Dr Webb had visited Linda's flat on many occasions for domiciliary consultations. 'How could you keep a tortoise there? Tortoises like to roam. You have no garden. And why a tortoise?' I have also always been impressed, and often bemused, by the tenacious way in which a psychiatrist will pursue a line of questioning, no matter how bizarre or irrelevant.

'I thought it could roam in the kitchen,' replied Linda. 'And I bought it because John won't let me have a baby. That's what we'd been arguing about.' Dr Webb nodded; he understood. 'So what did John do?' Linda looked angry. Her eyes brimmed with tears. 'He walked out on me. I can never live when he walks out on me and so. . . and so. . . I took the slug pellets.' There followed a good deal of weeping and sniffing, interspersed with nose-blows, of some force, into paper tissues which we had each donated from our own pockets.

Until that point, my contribution to the proceedings had been minimal. Being conscious of this, I decided to interrupt her display of emotion. I asked, earnestly, 'What has become of the tortoise?' She dabbed her nose. 'No problem there,' she said. I relaxed, imagining that she had left a mound of lettuce for it to nibble through. 'After I'd taken the slug pellets, I threw it out of the window.'

Two questions immediately leapt into my mind upon receipt of this disturbing information: 1. Why had Linda not offered the slug pellets to the tortoise and then jumped out of the window herself? 2. Had anyone been killed by the flying tortoise? It must have been an odd way to die, being poleaxed by a meteorite with four little legs and a quizzical expression.

Wisely, I said nothing.

The silence was broken by Dr Webb's sharp intake of breath; he rubbed his hands together. This was a sign that it was time for our conference. We left Linda, explaining that we would return in a few minutes. She greeted our departure with the same threat that had welcomed our arrival.

We peered up and down the ward's narrow entrance corridor, looking for a room where we might discuss Linda in private. Nowhere seemed suitable: the nurses' office was subject to repeated interruptions, the doctors' room contained two housemen who scribbled furiously in between answering their bleeps, and the patients' day-room was lined with elderly patients in armchairs dozing in front of a television screen upon which an Asian lady explained, at length, the correct way to approach chicken tikka masala. We stood uncomfortably in the corridor, waiting for a nurse to offer assistance; unfortunately, they were adhering to their policy of smirking and ignoring us. In desperation, Dr Webb ushered me into a small room with a sliding door, just adjacent to the nurses' office. Once inside, it became apparent that this room was, in fact, no more than a cupboard. It contained shelves of pillows and linen. There was nowhere to sit but it offered privacy, which Dr Webb regarded as vital for these discussions. The last thing I saw before he slid the door shut was Linda's face, peering from the entrance to her room. Her expression changed, just before her features were obliterated by the door, from curiosity to confusion.

My consultant turned to me. We were about to embark on a familiar discussion, assessing the pros and cons of various therapeutic options, when something in the way the door shut rendered us speechless. We stared at each other open-mouthed. The sliding of the door had been followed by an ominous and final click. It had locked. We had come to assess

a suicidal patient but we had achieved only self-incarceration.
We were two psychiatrists locked in a cupboard.

Neither of us wished to state the obvious. I was aware that
we were fast approaching a state of high farce. The sheen of
respect and gravity I liked to reserve for Dr Webb was
becoming difficult to maintain under the circumstances. He
exhaled slowly, then said, 'I think we have a problem.' As
ever, I felt I had little to contribute. 'Yes,' I said, nodding
hard.

He knocked feebly at the door and proferred a small cry of,
'excuse me.' He repeated this, slightly louder. It was difficult
to reconcile the need to draw attention to ourselves without
actually drawing attention to ourselves. It was clear why
Linda's expression had changed to confusion, perhaps even
amusement. She had known this was a cupboard. In my
mind, the scene became a split screen. On one side was
Linda, manipulating the situation. On the other, us,
imprisoned psychiatrists, pummelling pathetically on the
immovable door.

'My psychiatrists have locked themselves in a cupboard,'
wailed Linda.

We heard this and it was enough to arrest our attack on the
door; we listened intently. I could envisage those smirking
nurses' disbelief turning to panic. How, they wondered,
would Linda react to this grotesque insult? What impulse
would take her? With what self-administered poison, would
she protest? They would be descending on her with a verbal
straitjacket: 'There, there, it's OK, they won't be gone long,
we'll get you a nice cup of tea. . .' Meanwhile, potentially
harmful objects would be stealthily removed from her room:
the cord round the dressing gown, the cutlery, the stagnant
water in the vase of flowers. While they smothered her in
attention and rendered her room harmless, their accomplices
would be searching frantically for the key.

On our side of the screen, we shuffled impatiently. For
want of anything more useful to do, I knocked again on the
door and was startled to hear a voice reciprocate. 'The key,'
it said, loudly and clearly. 'We can't find the key.' I turned
to Dr Webb and said, a little unnecessarily, 'they can't find
the key.' It was then, in turning to face him, that I noticed the

window. It was small, and difficult to reach, but it represented hope. To my surprise, Dr Webb accepted the idea; clearly, being locked in a cupboard for any great length of time had not featured prominently in his day's agenda. With the aid of the shelves, I climbed up to the window, forced it open and, with a look which I hoped transmitted comradeship but undoubtedly betrayed fear, I tumbled through. With a twist and a lurch, I was free. Moments later, I stood on a small lawned area outside the medical ward, repositioning my tie, which had come adrift during my exertions. I awaited events.

There was a very long pause punctuated only by a number of grunts from the other side of the window. I made noises which I hoped were encouraging. It was at this point that the full comical force of the situation started to overwhelm me. A smile developed on my face and continued broadening as Dr Webb's buttocks came into view. For some reason, he had decided to reverse out of the window. Suppressed laughter caused a tension in my abdomen, not unlike unrelieved flatulence. I was edging my way towards an abyss of helpless hysterics.

His bottom was in full view now. In a nearby glass-fronted corridor, two domestics, each with mop and bucket, stood observing us. Dr Webb's bottom wriggled more desperately. I lurched nearer the abyss.

Noises suggesting great exertion emanated from where I imagined Dr Webb's head to be. Then there was a groan and, significantly, the bottom wriggling stopped. He was stuck. His shortly portly buttocks were furious. 'Get us down from here,' they snarled. 'We're busy.' The domestics continued to stare.

I realized that some sort of intervention was required, so, with a cheery reassuring platitude, I grasped the few folds of his jacket that had come into view. Face to cheek with his astonishing and astonished bottom, I tugged and he writhed. I wondered if I should fetch some forceps. I was reminded of a tortoise, perhaps Linda's tortoise, desperately attempting the impossible: to escape from its own shell. Then, quite suddenly, we were a heap of red faces and crumpled clothes sitting on the grass.

I smiled thinly as I searched for something appropriate to say. It was then that it happened. In the distance, in the glass-fronted corridor, I noticed the two domestics. One had turned to the other. It was too far for me to hear or even to lip read, yet, somehow, I knew with absolute certainty what had been said. She had made a comment by way of explanation to her partner, who bore a puzzled expression. This is what she said: 'It's OK – they're psychiatrists.' Both then gave a half nod and a look of complete acceptance and understanding. Then they resumed mopping the floor.

I teetered and then plummeted into the abyss. I was helpless. The pretence of self-control, the vestige of dignity evaporated as I gave vent to howls of laughter. Dr Webb, to his credit, smiled. And waited. We had no tissues with which to wipe my tears – Linda had used our supply. So I wiped my face on my jacket sleeve. The whole process of hysterics, exhaustion, recovery and drying off took about five minutes. Dr Webb, still smiling, remained patient. 'OK?' he asked finally. 'OK,' I said.

We walked to the glass corridor, past the domestics, who deemed it unnecessary to look up from their mopping, and returned to the medical ward. We stood in the ward entrance. The nursing staff had disappeared, probably surrounding and imploring Linda who at that point, I imagined, was standing on her chair, threatening to jump. Two burly and giggling porters stood outside the cupboard door, poised with what looked like a large hammer and chisel. These were men who obviously had a funny story to tell; they decided to tell us.

'Guess what we've got in here?' asked one, smiling. 'Two psychiatrists!' exclaimed his partner, with evident glee. 'Two psychiatrists who've locked themselves in a cupboard,' elucidated the first. 'I can't wait to see their faces when we let them out!' And then they set about demolishing the door.

Dr Webb turned to me. 'Let's come back after lunch,' he said.

KEITH HOPCROFT
Basildon

Ballads of Bad Habits

Her Song

Oh my love, he has a red red nose,
  His liver's out of tune,
Oh my love, he's lost his memory,
  Can't tell July from June.
As ill art thou, my fuddled friend,
  So deep in debt am I,
And we'll both go downhill, my dear,
  Until ye can gang dry.

Until ye can gang dry, my dear
  And the bottle ye can shun:
We'll have to rob the till, my dear
  When out of cash we run.
So steel your will, my only love
  And take your pills awhile
Cos if you drink again, my love
  I'll run ten thousand mile.

His Song

Drink to me only with thine eyes
  And I the pledge will sign
Put antabuse into my cup
  And spirits I'll decline.
The thirst I now must exorcise
  My health did undermine,
And now my ulcer plays me up
  If I touch beer or wine.
The ills my drinking did bequeath
  Have forced me to agree
My liver is the worse for wear
  Sky high my GGT
The whisky-tainted fumes I breathe
  Have caused my love to flee
And 'brewer's droop', I do declare,
  The final straw for me.

The Doctor's Song

Beautiful dreamer, last century
Laudanum and bromide were fashioned for thee,
Fearing insomnia spoiling the night,
Drugged to the eyeballs you'd turn out the light.
  Beautiful dreamer, surely 'twas wrong
  Seeking your solace in this remedy,
  Still, when barbiturates came along
  Beautiful dreamer, you grasped them with glee.

Beautiful dreamer, as time goes by,
You look for something more modern to try,
Mandrax is next, till law intervenes,
Then come the benzodiazepines.
  Beautiful dreamer, open you eyes,
  You keep demanding these tablets from me;
  When you got hooked, and you feign surprise,
  Beautiful dreamer, don't blame your GP.

The Patient's Reply

Here I lie while sleep eludes me
  All through the night.
Still the land of dreams excludes me
  All through the night.
Through the endless hours it's boring
Listening to my partner's snoring
For some respite I'm imploring
  All through the night.
At the doctor's clinic waiting
  'Til late at night,
Not much use anticipating
  Help with my plight.
He thinks my complaints are fiction
Reads me lectures on addiction
Unconcerned for my affliction
All through the night.

Now it's 2am I'll call him
  Out in the night.
Though the prospect may appal him
  This time of night.
Since his manner's so uncaring
My insomnia he'll be sharing
Then he'll know why I'm despairing
  All through the night.

MARIE CAMPKIN
London

Rhubarb, Rhubarb

For years I thought it was just a personal fad, but now I realize that it's an illness and I share it with many sufferers. I just hope by publicizing that it's a phobia and we can't help it, a sizeable slice of mankind may eventually obtain some relief from their misery.

And who are we unfortunates? We are the rhubarbophobics, that's who; the people who have to smile and bear it as the rest of humanity shovels rhubarb jam, rhubarb tarts, rhubarb custard, rhubarb fool and a host of other rhubarb unmentionables at us.

Maybe there was a time in my life when I liked rhubard but, if so, the recollection has gone. Much of my boyhood was during World War II when rationing was severe and any kind of fruit was a delicacy. Scotland, where I grew up, has a short summer: its fruits are delicious but their season is brief.

Except for blasted rhubarb, that is. I liked apples, doted on brambles and adored raspberries and strawberries, yet they would come and go in a winking. But rhubarb was forever. The moment there was even the faintest thought of spring in the air, these ominous, crinkly, dark-green leaves began to push up through the soil, and soon the pink stalks beneath them were turning bright red.

It seemed no time before us children were being fed the ghastly stuff, and it's so prolific that friends and relatives would bring armfuls of it when they came to visit, saying stupid things like, 'We know the young 'uns love the stuff'. I only knew a couple of kids my age who actually liked it, and they've probably died ages ago of cumulative rhubarb poisoning since the rest of us were so keen to offload our supplies on them.

One of these aberrant infants used to eat it raw, like celery, and his parents would give up some of their precious sugar ration so that he could dip the end of the stalk in it. With the combined assault of sucrose and rhubarbic acid, all his teeth fell out before he was ten.

I grew up trying to avoid rhubarb, but it came to me from all directions. I formed the strongest impression that it was forced on youngsters because the grown-ups wouldn't touch the ghastly stuff themselves and I resolved that when I was adult I would never eat it again. And then I married and in doing so made only one mistake.

My wife is all but perfect and I stand by that view after many years of marriage except – and it's a very big except – she loves rhubarb and so, throughout my married life I've been eating the stuff with a smile, (actually, on reflection, it's not a smile, it's an involuntary rictus brought on by the rhubarb's sourness which no sweetener can hide from my discerning palate), and, each spring, watching with horror as it regularly reappears in our garden, spreading a little more and a little more.

I've dropped hints, I've occasionally spoken my mind, I've even thrown the odd tantrum or two. I've 'accidentally' dug up the rhubarb plot on at least one occasion and, in feigned ignorance, once mowed it with the lawnmower. My wife looked – and was – hurt, but the rhubarb apparently wasn't and shot up even healthier as soon as my back was turned.

Then, two years ago, my neighbour did some massive landscaping in his garden and, by inadvertence (I call it an Act of God) the contractor totally buried our rhubarb bed in

tons of rubble, top soil and bark chips. We had no more
rhubarb that summer and, bliss! no rhubarb appeared at all
last year. And so began tentative, tremulous hopes that, at
last. . .

But no, this spring, before the snowdrops, the crocuses or
the daffodils had appeared, there was a great heaving of oak
chips and rocks and, all over the place, the dreaded leaflets
were pushing up. The thought occurs that it's Zombie
rhubarb, risen from the dead to haunt me and, if so, there's
every chance it'll taste even viler than before.

ALISTAIR MUNRO
Canada

Night Terrors

L et me start by saying that psychiatry has never been my
strong point. In fact, if I were to be perfectly honest, I'd
have to admit that I know less about psychiatry than about
any other speciality in medicine. Don't misunderstand me. I
can give anorexics back their appetites and badger bulimiacs
out of binging with the best of them. I can provide the paper
hankies for my depressed tearful female patients as well as
anyone else. I can even let them pour out their troubles for
hours on end. My receptionists tell me I'm too caring. My
partners tell me I'm too soft. But when it comes to someone
who is really unbalanced, then I have to admit I call in the
experts. Day or night, even on the weekend, I'll track them
down. I'll chase them through as many answerphone links as
they care to provide, and eventually get them in. Much better
for the patient, and much more reassuring for me.

I guess I could write all I know about psychiatry on the back
of a postage stamp. I blame it on the fact that our psychiatry
block was just before Christmas. You can't expect immature
medical students to choose boring old psychiatry clinics in
preference to the opportunity to complete the Christmas
shopping, and enjoy all those parties. It was one of the best
Christmas periods I remember. Which is just my way of

choosing to rationalize my total inability to assess Mrs
Meredith in her true colours, until it was far too late. To be
fair, my partners had dealt with her too, so they were no
better. But it wasn't they who nearly came to a very sticky
end that cold dark night in December. It was I.

She was proving to be one of our most troublesome
alcoholic patients, these days. Here I was again, parted from
my wonderful warm bed at 3am, driving down the bumpy,
dark lane, just to reassure her about some stupid hypo-
chondriacal problem, more than likely. As I struggled to see
through the driving rain, I wondered what law of nature
makes it always rain when I am on call. Is it only me that
suffers this fate – are there other GPs on whom Lady Luck
smiles benignly? Do they always have fine weather and
sunshine to cheer them through their time on call? As my
mind wanders off in this way, I pull myself together, and for
perhaps the thousandth time as I drive through such a night,
I worry about the dangers of sleep deprivation, and promise
myself early nights for the remainder of the week.

At 3am, driving round the countryside, there is a certain
seductiveness surrounding sleep. At 9pm the next night,
seated comfortably in front of the television, the whole sleep
deprivation thing seems much less important. But here, in
the middle of this foul night, I find myself honestly
wondering if all this lack of sleep is having some permanent
effect on my brain.

I'd been a bit suspicious recently when I'd visited Mrs
Meredith; she'd seemed more confused than actually drunk.
Very distant, very vague, as if she couldn't understand my
words. Only 50 years old, after all, even though she looked
double; she seemed to be acting very strangely sometimes,
almost as if she was talking to someone else that I couldn't
see. Just the alcohol, I suppose, knocking-off the grey cells.
Still, might be worth asking the 'Trick Cyclists' to see her
anyway, just in case.

Funny how I still think of psychiatrists by my old partner's
nickname for them. I guess I heard him call them that a
hundred times, and somehow it has stuck. Maybe I'm going
a bit senile myself, with all these disturbed nights. My brain
not getting enough rest to renew its own grey cells. I'm still

worrying about my mental capabilities, as I bump my way to
the end of the deserted lane, and park the car. Getting out of
the car, I inadvertently get my bag stuck in a bush. I never
really find a good place to park, even when I'm doing house
calls in the daytime. Always a puddle, dog's droppings, a
pot-hole, or a quagmire, ready to receive my dainty size
3 stiletto. Shivering, I rip my bag free, uprooting some shrub
or other. Staggering over the uneven pathway, in the black-
ness, I wonder with a somewhat cynical smile whether it is
me that's really drunk, not my patient. Sensing someone
watching me from the shadows, I spin round, sweat breaking
out on the back of my neck. Momentarily I am mesmerized
by the brightness of a neighbourhood cat's eyes. Instantly I
am transported back to this very lane one day last summer.
I can see it all so clearly: the moggy monster curled up asleep
on the warm bonnet of my car when I returned from yet
another unnecessary visit to Mrs Meredith. When it refused
to be dislodged by a few jerky steering manoeuvres, (other
people call it a three point turn), I got out and tried to scoop
it gently off the bonnet. It took exception, and sunk its tabby
teeth into my hand. I can still see the entire pratice staff trying
to control their laughter when I returned and related my tale,
and of course the Practice Nurse couldn't contain her desire
to use up the last tetanus booster in my behind. Don't be
silly, this is probably a different cat entirely, I rationalize,
stepping carefully past it all the same, resisting the temptation to use my case to push it out of the way anyway. The
house is in darkness. The rain pours down. No one deigns to
answer my urgent attack on the door. 'So what's new,' I
mutter, pushing hard against the door, and eventually
heaving it open halfway. My mutter changes to a yelp as I
crack my shin against the hall table, sweeping it before me as
I head for the staircase. I stumble around for some time
before I eventually find the lightswitch, and replace the
probably priceless potpourri dish back on the table, minus
most of its contents. Lit only by a 40 watt bulb, the hallway
looks different tonight – sort of spooky somehow. That's
enough of that silliness, I remonstrate silently with myself as
I start the long climb.

I am halfway up the first flight of stairs before it dawns on
me exactly what is different downstairs. Usually the light is

on in the hallway, and her husband is sitting smoking his pipe behind a newspaper in the room on the right. Totally unwilling to get involved in his wife's management, as I found to my disbelief on my very first night visit here. Nothing to do with him, he'd declared, still with his pipe in his mouth, poking through a convenient gap in his carious teeth. I had left him in peace ever since. But he was always there whatever time of the day or night. Until tonight. How strange.

No point wasting my breath shouting to ask where she is – she's always in the very top bedroom. As I toil up the final staircase, I wish I'd kept up my Jane Fonda exercise regime, or at least kept myself a bit fitter. Grabbing the banister and heaving myself up the last couple of steps, I can see the light under her bedroom door. As I push open the door, she is already rambling, clutching a whisky bottle to her chest. As I enter, the ramblings gain volume but not much else. 'He didn't deserve it. . . I shouldn't have done it. . . He was a good man. . . I loved him, even if he did call me a drunk. . ., she broke off into a wailing sound that made me think of banshees, and ghost stories. The bedroom was in an even greater state of disarray than usual, as if there had been some kind of struggle. There was a very strong smell of something decidedly unpleasant too. Maybe I could get the Environmental Health people to intervene and have her removed from our patch.

She was still rambling on. I supposed I'd better try to find out the latest problem, if I was to have any chance of catching up on some sleep before morning surgery. 'OK Mrs Meredith. Stop that noise and tell me what the problem is. Then we can both get back to sleep.' 'In the wardrobe. . . look in the wardrobe. . . I shouldn't have done it. . . I loved him. . . honestly doctor, I didn't mean it, but he made me so angry. . .' This didn't seem to be getting us anywhere. 'Tell me what it is about your husband that's upsetting you.'

As I said it, I remembered that my junior partner had mentioned a few days ago that he thought her husband had finally walked out. When my partner had visited, he'd thought her decidedly odd, and muttering strangely about her husband. When challenged, she would only say that he had gone. And here she was, several days later, still apparently in the same distraught state as before. She must have really cared about the guy, despite the way she treated him. So that explained why the downstairs hall was all in darkness tonight. Imagine what it must be like to be here all alone in this mausoleum of a house, though. Little wonder she had invited me to visit her tonight. Maybe this was the start of even worse days to come. Heaving a sigh, I attempted to concentrate on the present, and her largely incoherent ramblings. Through her hysteria, she kept gesturing toward the wardrobe. 'Open the door and you'll see what I've done. I shouldn't have done it. . . I really did love him. . . in the wardrobe. . .' The wailing started even louder this time, as if to prompt me to do what she wanted and look in the wardrobe.

She really did look a bit mad tonight, with that glazed look in her eyes. Yes, I'd get the specialist out to see her first thing in the morning, see what an expert would think. Of course, in the morning chances are she would seem much less frightening anyway, but at least I would rest easy in my bed at night, knowing that I had done all that I could to help her get better. And perhaps if they took her into hospital and tried to dry her out, we would have a respite from the calls. My car suspension would certainly welcome the holiday, even if I did lose out on a few night visit fees. But first I supposed I'd better do as I was told, and look in this damn wardrobe. Decisively, I spun round and grabbed the door handle, then stopped in my tracks as I felt an icy chill of horror grip me. It all fell into place. Her husband's disappearance, her terrified and almost mad look, her desire for me to look in the wardrobe. And that overpowering smell of rotting flesh. And me, all seven stone of me, stuck here with the murderer in the middle of the night, on the top floor of an otherwise empty house, at the bottom of a deserted lane. I spun round again, deciding instantly that I was not going to look in any wardrobe without half the country's police force beside me. I had just decided that making a run for it was perhaps the safest course in the circumstances, until I turned for the door and found her standing in front of it.

'Never let a psychiatric patient get between you and the door' the professor had thundered. It was the only thing I remembered from my whole psychiatry block as a student.

I had never really understood the advice until now. Somehow it didn't look like I was getting out of that room until I had looked in the wardrobe. And she was now brandishing the whisky bottle, rather than clutching it.

'I didn't like your attitude last time you were here, doctor. Don't upset me again. I won't tolerate it this time. It's because of you that I did it.' No rambling now. With sickening clarity I too remembered my last visit to her about a week ago. What awful thing had I unintentionally made her do, I wondered, already sure of the answer. Angry with her repeated suicide attempts and persisting alcohol abuse, despite my attempts to reform her, I had warned her of the way ahead if she chose not to stop. It had been a stormy and acrimonious consultation, which had ended with her almost throwing me out. I had felt pretty shaken up afterwards, certain that violence might have ensued if her husband hadn't stopped her from chasing me through the entrance hall. It seemed my feelings had been right, judging by the way the whisky bottle was raised above her head now. And her poor husband in no position to intervene this time. I shuddered. Suddenly it felt very cold in the room. 'Look in the wardrobe, see what I've done.' This time it was a command. The whisky bottle went higher. I could feel it's hardness in my mind, as I envisaged it cracking it's way through my occiput. Fear clutched my heart; sweat trickled down my spine. If I discovered her husband's fate, would I be the next?

I closed my eyes, muttered a quick prayer, and opened them to find that the whisky bottle had been magically replaced by a breadknife which must have been hidden in her dressing gown. The glorious technicolour picture in my mind changed. Now I could see myself lying in a pool of blood, with the dead body from the wardrobe slumped on top of me. I could even see the headline in the local paper 'Knifed on Night Call – Doctor in Death Drama'. Well, it seemed my fate was set. As she started to gesture towards the wardrobe again, this time with the knife, I felt the time had come to take my chance, and open the box. Very slowly, I turned my back on her, while a voice inside me screamed the professor's instructions never to turn your back on a psychiatric patient. Easing the door slowly open, I let out a

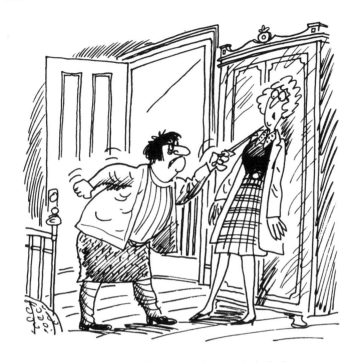

Sue moved even closer to my throat with the knife.

scream, as something soft fell against my legs, and sunk it's teeth into my ankle. That damn cat again. Simultaneously I felt, rather than saw, the source of the dreadful smell, as my right foot squelched into the parcel of cat poo which had fallen out of the wardrobe. I only glimpsed the disarray inside before slamming the door again. I had a mental picture of her husband's suits and trousers slashed to shreds, presumably by the very weapon she was now wielding too close to my right shoulder blade. So that was all she had done.

Tears of relief poured down my face; stupid really since, as I turned, she moved even closer to my throat with the knife. 'It's all right Mrs Meredith. I'm not angry with you. It will all be all right.' Even to my ears I sounded terrified, rather than reassuring. How stupid and placatory could I be. How could I stand here in the middle of the night, and say everything would be wonderful, when a complete nutcase was standing not two inches from my carotids with a breadknife. And she had obviously had plenty of practise using it, judging by the contents of the wardrobe. I was frightened to swallow too hard in case I should be treated to a very amateur tracheostomy. How I wished I'd gone to those psychiatry lectures, now. Suddenly I would have given anything to go back and sit through even the most boring sessions. I suppose this whole experience was some long-delayed divine retribution. Struggling to remain calm, I opened my mouth to try some more conciliatory comments. But nothing would come out. It was like one of those dreadful nightmares where you wake up trying to scream, but no sound will come. I cleared my throat. Tried again. Still absolutely nothing. Somehow it didn't seem appropriate to smile as I thought how pleased my husband or even my partners would be if I'd actually been struck dumb permanently. How they would love it.

Terrified to move anything except my eyes, I looked around desperately for something to use to defend myself. Her mad, glazed eyes followed mine. 'Don't try anything silly'. Still cold and in command. No sign of the confused ramblings now, except from me. It seemed my only chance was to try and entice her away from her stance in front of the bedroom door, then take a chance that I'd be faster on my feet down those three flights of stairs. As I transferred my weight slowly onto my other foot, in preparation, I winced as I remembered the damage inflicted by her crazy cat. How on earth could I sprint down the stairs wounded and in pain. She reach towards the whisky bottle where it had fallen onto the floor. I saw my opportunity, waited until she was off-balance, and pushed her sideways. I was through the door, and halfway across the landing before I was aware of her too close behind me for comfort.

'Stop' she commanded. My stupid feet did exactly as she said, while my body continued its progress. I measured my length on the top landing. She towered over me, rambling once more, then in an almost drunken stagger, she lurched forward, narrowly missing me with the knife, and stabbed herself through the diaphragm in some hideous attempt at 'hara kiri'.

Fighting back the nausea, and still a trifle wary that this was just some kind of plot to throw me off my guard, I felt for her carotid pulse and confirmed it was still there. Shaking, I started back towards the staircase, limping and leaving a trail of feline faeces behind me. Suddenly, the old house really frightened me. Shadows were everywhere, despite turning on every light I could find. I'm not sure why, since I believed we were alone in the house, but I kept looking over my shoulder. Did I honestly expect the victim to rise again and chase after me, like in the video nasties I refuse to watch on television? Did I expect skeletons in the shadows, and corpses cluttering up cupboards? How could I possibly have marched in here so many times before, in the dark, blasé about this spooky house, and its occupants? Would tonight teach me caution or only terror and trepidation? Would night calls ever be the same again? Eventually I found the telephone in the corner of her husband's room. And still no sign of him. I stood there momentarily mesmerized by the events of the last half-hour. Who should I call? Reminding myself that there had in fact been no murder, to the best of my knowledge anyway, I chose Ambulance Control. They said later that I sounded a trifle strange that night, as I requested an urgent ambulance for a stabbing.

I left the wardrobe doors closed as I waited for the ambulance to arrive. The boys were more upset by the three flights of stairs when they did arrive than by how I had come to witness this bizarre suicide attempt or why I threw myself into their arms crying like a baby. With their usual calm unhurried manner, they provided paper hankies for me, oxygen for my victim and safe transportation down the lane without so much as a single bump for the breadknife. Suddenly, I was alone again, fighting with the bushes and scrambling back into the safety of my car, as the bleep blared out. Life goes on.

I'm not sure how I appeared at the next house. Somewhat dishevelled, I suspect, but it didn't seem to bother them, so long as I got granny into hospital with her heart attack.

Driving home, it all seemed unreal. I found myself wondering again if sleep deprivation was doing something to my brain. Was I having some sort of strange night terrors while driving around the countryside? And if in the morning I should find out it was all real – how to explain to my husband who needs ten hours sleep a night, that from now on, night calls will have to involve him as chaperone. I struggled into bed at 5am. My husband didn't stir. I was still worried it was all a dream. I couldn't bring myself to waken him. I was still awake when the alarm went off. I thought I'd better share my story. He laughed, confirmed I'd been dreaming. I was reassured for my patient's sake, but thought I'd better book that psychiatrist for myself.

I didn't tell my partners. Halfway through morning surgery, the local general surgeon 'phoned to confirm that he had managed to save my patient. She had just been sectioned and would be transferred to the local funny farm at the earliest opportunity. A surgical ward with its array of sharp instruments did not seem the appropriate place to keep her for longer than absolutely necessary. I wasn't sure whether to be relieved, or relive my terror.

My partners seemed a little put out by the story. We agreed to take her off our list. I worked the day as usual, despite protestations from my partners that I should go home and recover.

Interestingly, her husband was never heard of again in the village. We heard he never visited her in hospital. Even now, as I venture out on some dark nights, and drive pass the end of her lane, I still shudder, as I remember that night, and wonder. . . You see, I never really looked properly in that wardrobe. He might still be there, sacrificed along with his suits.

PAMELA M. R. BROWN
Swansea

Anna Bollics

I've not come about my sister, doc,
Though look what happened to him.
He used to be known as Jane, doc,
Now everyone knows her as Jim.

They said it would build her up, doc,
Save hours of work in the gym.
Have muscles of steel like Rambo, doc,
That's what they said to him.

She never had much of a bust, doc,
She said that she liked being slim,
But at least you could tell which was front, doc,
If ever she went for a swim.

She took these weird looking tabs, Doc,
The effects were startling and grim,
He's happy enough, it's me that is sick,
I've had it right up to the brim.

RICHARD WYNDHAM
Marlingford

The Fitting Munchausen

One Tuesday night, when Pete and Tom were house surgeons in a large Glasgow hospital, they admitted a man in the early morning as he appeared to have renal colic but had about eight operation scars across his abdomen. However, the situation was complicated by the fact that the man appeared to be deaf and dumb. They communicated with written messages and as the ward was full, they placed him in a bed at the door of the ward. During the night, the man became very restless and so cot-sides were put up on the bed. Just after eight in the morning, they were called from their bedrooms which were adjacent to the ward, as the man had become very aggressive. They tried to calm him and wrote a message for him asking him to be quiet for half an hour: the senior consultant was a caring surgeon and always came in early on the Wednesday morning to assess the patients of the night. This man became quite violent and having beckoned a nurse over, he then struck her in the face with his clenched fist. This was too much for Pete who then stunned the patient with a blow to the chin. Just then the consultant walked in to the ward and reacted angrily to the scene. He ordered Pete and Tom away from the bed, went up to the patient and asked sister for the pad and pencil. He handed these to the patient who wrote a message and returned the pad. The bed was soon being wheeled to the ward door and the patient forcibly dressed as he had written on the pad: 'F _ _ _ off, I am waiting for the big white chief.'

Some three years later, Pete was registrar in a hospital in London and was called to casualty as there was a man having major fits and it seemed that he could not speak. As he entered the department, Pete paused to observe the scene. On the floor was a man who appeared to be having fits and was whirling round the floor with his feet lashing out. Strangely, he only seemed to kick nurses legs and never hit his legs on a trolley. There was something familiar about the man so Pete approached and with help managed to get a look at his abdomen. Sure enough, there were numerous scars and as the staff now told him that the man was deaf and dumb, he realized it was the same man as he had encountered in Glasgow. He took the pad that the nurses had been using and wrote on it. 'Remember me from Glasgow? Well you f _ _ _ off now.' The man was up and away in a shot leaving behind only his description in the casualty 'Black Book'.

JOHN A. J. MACLEOD
Western Isles

Stream of Consciousness

'You want me to see a psychiatrist, doc? I mean to say they're just chaps who ask a lot of expensive questions my wife would ask for nothing. I've this problem, see: I can't figure out where I finish off and everyone else begins. It's the same with any speciality these days. I got insured with BUPA and that. Now you want me to see one of these mind-benders and that goes on my record, see. BUPA or whoever it is will have me on their records as having had to see a psychiatrist. How's that going to look, eh? You know how it is with the mind, doc; it's one way traffic through the till. Six weeks in the bin for starters. Mind you – I've heard the food is very good and there might be some decent birds there. Oops! There I go again. You know, doc, there's nothing quite like the thrill I get when holding the door open for a feminist. I don't believe they think they're women as such; but there it is – a psychiatrist, eh? Who'd have thought I'd come to this? Its's a bit of a come-down after a life at the top. Anyway – what's his game, eh? I mean – what's he going to do to me? I suppose he has penetrating eyes; well I'll bloody well stare back at him. Two can play at that game. What's that you said? Yuh – I'm sure he's very clever. Who ever met a doctor who wasn't clever? It's one thing to be clever and quite another to be intelligent – and there's me; just plain lucky for all my life. And now this. Why? Just because I don't happen to think the same as any one else you think I need help; that's it, isn't it? I like being the way I am. I'm doing no one any harm. Anyway – what's a fellah doing sitting in a chair all day and seeing people like me? What was that? OK – so there's no one like me. I assume you meant that as an insult – what? – a compliment; well – thanks for nothing. Yuh – I know I need a bath. Being dirty is a way of life but I've kept healthier than most. I mean – you don't get to sleep rough every night without getting hardened up a bit – know what I mean? When I leave your office, doc, there won't be a damp patch on your precious chair – it wouldn't take a genius to spot the layers of paper you put on the chair before I came in. I'm not as dirty as I look, you know. No – you can't deny it. Don't tell me you put down fresh paper for each new patient. Spare me that, doc. Anyway – what is a Day Hospital?'

JAMES HENRY PITT-PAYNE
Beckenham

The Changing Face of Psychiatry

'Lock them up and throw away the key!' Not so very long ago this was the treatment for the mentally disturbed. Only the most docile patients could expect 'community care'. They became village idiots. Nowadays we are more democratic. Village idiots are elected and we have psychiatrists.

The old asylums, once walled enclaves outside the city gates, have sunk into suburbia. Their grounds have been sold off and the hospital farms have sprouted homogeneous houses. These new estates probably consume more tranquillizers per acre than the madhouse ever did.

British hospitals tore down their perimeter walls long before the idea caught on in Berlin.

'We are now an open-door hospital,' the administrator proudly announced. He then handed over a large bunch of keys. Unfortunately, the staff shortage meant that the patients still had to be locked in. But there was an open-door, policy! When is a door not a door?

While hospitals have become physically more open, it can be difficult to admit an acutely disturbed patient. Searching for the duty psychiatrist can be a tedious task. No longer men in white coats, they seem to blend in with their patients! The GP may have to dangle the carrot of the specialist domicilary visit fee. A certain Dr. Smith did so many domicilary visits he became known as D.V. Smith. In time, nobody remembered his real name!

Another obstacle the GP may need to overcome is the social work report. Admission may be difficult if the social worker believes that doctors are bourgeois lackeys of a capitalist system. 'Doctor! My client is not mad, because he believes MI5 are spying on him and beaming rays from his toaster. To send him to a mental hospital is a gross infringement of his civil liberties!'

I suppose admitting patients with hallucinations has always been tricky. Nobody got Joan of Arc into hospital when she heard voices. Look what happened to her!

Treatments have also changed. Once upon a time every hospital had a pet mosquito. This malaria carrying insect was used to treat syphilis. If a dose of quartan fever did not fix those spirochaetes, there was always the alternative therapy of arsenic! Drilling holes in the head, to let out the demons, was a medieval practice. It is now a medical practice called leucotomy.

Shock treatment (ECT for non-tabloid readers) used to be administered without anaesthetic. Patients were frozen, overdosed with insulin and given all sorts of bizarre remedies. No wonder some people got better. If you stayed in hospital for those treatments you had to be mad.

I often wonder how many of our NHS treatments of today will be ridiculed next century? As a psychiatric patient once said to me, 'The NHS is a great institution, but not everyone wants to live in an institution!'

JOHN STUART DOWDEN
Australia

Some Nervous Nursery Rhymes

Mental Health Act 1983

I had a little nut case
Nothing would she wear
But a silver G-string
And her golden hair.
Her husband and daughter
Came to visit me
And begged me to take
Her on Section Three.
I felt that I ought to
I said I'd agree.
But all the social workers
Wouldn't back me.

The Worm Turns

O dear what can the matter be?
John's gone mad as a hatter, he
Keeps on saying he'll batter me
    Thinks that I've had an affair.

When first we were courting he plied me with roses,
Liked taking my picture in artistic poses,
He used to come round with a bunch of blue ribbons
To tie up my bonny brown hair.

Now it's O dear what can the matter be?
I try teasing and flattery,
But if I start to natter, he
    Tells me I'd better beware.

  Now when he gets jealous he gets so dramatic,
  He threatens to lock me upstairs in the attic,
  He keeps bringing out this great bunch of blue ribbons
  And tying me down to the chair.

So it's O dear what can the matter be?
While I'm ragged and tattery
John gets fitter and fatter, he
    Soon will drive me to despair.

  I guess I suspected he was a bit kinky,
  But now he's gone potty and taken to drink, he
  May wake up and find himself stuffed with blue ribbons
  And hanging six feet in the air.

The Tower Block

Hush a bye baby, in the tower top,
When the wind gripes, your screaming won't stop –
When your Mum breaks, and lets baby fall,
Then a case conference we will call.

MARIE CAMPKIN
London

Stress Clinics

Stress clinics take place every Monday evening. They enable time to be spent on the anxious or mildly depressed person. A little while ago I had a visit from a chap who is rarely seen at the surgery. He was smartly dressed in a suit and had a Rotary Club badge in his lapel. He looked downcast. After the usual informalities, I asked him the matter. 'I feel depressed. I cannot cope. I have a burden on my mind and I wake early with black thoughts about the future.'

'How's your family?' I remembered they had three children and, although his wife did not work, she helped with meals on wheels and the local stroke club. Many years ago, she had all three children at home. I had been present at their births. 'Is it the job?', I asked. 'No, it's time. I'm busier than I have ever been.' He told me about the kinds of things he had to do, such as make people redundant, take difficult financial decisions and work long hours. From his tone and expressions, he had those things well under control. His mortgage on his house had been paid off. He had adequate money for luxuries.

'Do you have any hobbies?' 'Yes, I go shooting in the winter months. We have a shoot the other side of Coventry. Once a week. It's a great relaxation. I love the autumn and winter days in the open air'.

'Do you drink much?' 'Yes, lately, it helps me to relax'.

There was one last possibility.

'Do you have a girlfriend?' There was a pause. 'Yes,' he answered, then another long pause, 'two'.

I could not believe it. Here was a sexual Hercules of truly magnificent proportions.

'Two lovers and a wife?', I asked incredulously. 'Yes. I'm finding it difficult to cope.'

I did not know whether to shake him by the hand or condemn his morality. Sensible advice was needed.

'You will have to stop drinking and get yourself physically fit. You will need to loose two stone and take regular exercise. You remember what Shakespeare said about alcohol and lovermaking!'

He listened and smiled. He nodded in agreement.

To my surprise he followed my advice and even came to see me after six weeks. He looked a picture of health and happiness. He sat down in the chair and plopped a carrier bag down at his feet. I noticed a pheasant feather sticking out of the top.

I guessed he had brought me a gift of thanks. After the usual exchange of pleasantries, which told me he was better, he got up and handed me the bag.

'Here you are', he said with a broad grin, 'Hope you enjoy them, a brace of birds.'

JOHN SHENKMANS
Rugby

Cloud Cuckoo Land

Never tell anyone you're a doctor, apart from your patients and family who may have suspected anyway. Lie to the rest. Above all to travel agents. Two seconds of title-dropping in Paradise Suntours could ruin your holiday, particularly if you're flying. Airlines do not normally set aside two seats in Club class for the flight doctor to relax with his nurse after a busy surgery in the examination cubicle. Not even on long-haul flights. Especially on long-haul flights. Anyone who has ever felt ill while flying with 400 other holidaymakers to the Last Unspoilt Place on Earth will have discovered that medical facilities are in short supply. Briefly, there is no examination cubicle, no nurse and no doctor.

No doctor? Well, that depends. Your airline will have calculated that of 400 people who can afford to fly to the L.U.P.E on a £1500 package roughly five per cent will be medics. So, when the call goes up: 'Is there a doctor on board please?' and you have *Mr* Brown on your ticket, you must sit very tight. At the third call, when you realize the other nineteen doctors have also disowned their degrees, it's a struggle with your conscience.

My conscience is a bully and I am a coward. Putting down my large whiskey, I followed the steward to a very fat lady spread across two seats in the front row. I wasn't sure whether she started with two seats because of her size, or perhaps a sympathetic passenger had relinquished his. She was clearly having a panic attack and was hyperventilating frantically, stopping only briefly to tell me she could not breathe. My impression was that her problem was breathing too much so I found her a brown paper bag to breathe into. Her husband was unimpressed with this accepted but archaic-looking manoeuvre. 'She's a suspected heart case,

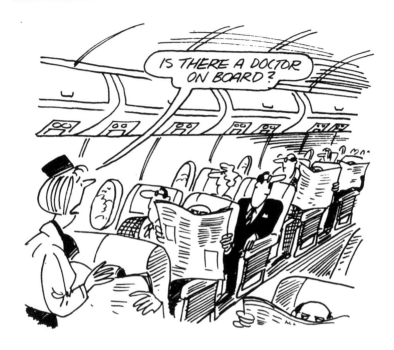

At the third call, when you realize the other nineteen doctors have also disowned their degrees. . . .

doctor. She has these attacks every time she flies. Are you a heart specialist?'

I was tempted to suggest that they would need to travel on Concorde to attract a volunteer cardiologist. He looked manic and started shaking. 'She needs a cardiograph, doctor.'

The steward reappeared with a sealed white box marked 'OPEN IN EMERGENCY'. I sensed the surrounding passengers challenging me to 'Open the box!' and since the husband was beginning to look quite ill by now, I declared an emergency and cut the seal, revealing a sphygmomanometer, a stethoscope, several elasticated bandages, and sticky plasters. This would have suited a hypertensive with a sprained ankle but not a suspected heart case. Meanwhile the husband fainted and banged his head on the box. His wife, who had now fully recovered, threw herself down beside him, stroked his brow and moaned endearments. As he came round I stuck a plaster on his forehead and she popped a Valium into his mouth.

'Are those yours or his?' I asked. 'Ours' she replied, as I returned to finish my whiskey, taking care to avoid the gaze of my other 398 patients.

P. J. SOUTH
Cranbrook

The Hell Centre

R arely does reading the address on an envelope bring a smile to the doctor's face, as well as giving a clue about the sender's diagnosis. Such was the case however with a letter my partner received from a depressed Irish Catholic lady. She had posted it to 'The Surgatory'.

If her condition deteriorates, I guess we can expect her to re-register with a Hell Centre.

T. G. STAMMERS
London

John

I have a lot of time for John. If I had to live with his wife I'd want to be on Ativan too. You know what it's like though; no GP worth his salt prescribes Ativan without delivering a short lecture entitled 'The perils of benzodiazepines.' You have it to do; it's part of the job description. When you join the College they make you roll up your left trouser-leg and swear that you'll never, ever prescribe Ativan without the lecture.

So here I am, giving John the lecture. Of course, I've given it every month for the last two years. Today, of course, is different; I'm really going to get through to him today. 'Now, look here, John, isn't it really time you thought about stopping these? I know times have been difficult, but I do think you could try and manage on two for a bit and then we could take it from there.' Something in my eyes perhaps, something in my voice?. . . 'OK, I'll give it a try. . .' Shock, horror, this has never happened before! What do I do now?

And he does give it a try, and he manages it. And three months later, he's down to one, then a half and he's off them in six months!

'John, this is wonderful, I'm really delighted.' 'Ay, well, I'm pleased meself,' he says, and looks shifty. I leave him alone.

'Well, John, what can I do for you today?' 'You can give me back them tablets, for a start. She's driving me round the bend. I don't get a moment's peace.' 'But, John, they're no answer, you can't give up like this. You did so well. . .' 'You don't know what she's like. She's up and down all night, can't sleep, can't stay still, and when she does go to sleep she gets nightmares and screams the place down. Then in the day she's a bag of nerves; weeping, shouting, I can't stand it. . .' 'But John, if she's that bad, why don't you get her to come and see me herself. There's not much point in treating you, when she's the one that's got the problem.' 'Well, she were fine on them tablets,' he shouts, then looks wildly at me. A long, embarrassed pause, then I said, 'What tablets, John?'

He'd been putting them in her tea, of course. I think at first he probably had taken them himself, but found soon enough that they worked better on her than him. We had quite a long chat and sorted it out, and I never saw his wife, but from what John said later, it took her a long time to get over the withdrawal.

ANDREW PROCTER
Gainsborough

Advanced Eccentricity

The literature in neuropsychiatry is surprisingly deficient in the commoner neural disorders I see in my practice. Take Mrs Katie for instance.

She drives into the surgery car park in a clapped-out Volkswagen Beetle and parks diagonally across two bays. A leg dressed in a mauve patterned stocking appears unsteadily out of the door followed by a full flowing caftan which is also mauve. It's her favourite colour.

There is always a striking hat. She must have a larder full because they usually have wax fruit on them. Today's is a black straw one with a brim about one and a half feet wide. It has satin flowers sewn to it. She suffers from one of my favourite diseases; advanced eccentricity. I collect them.

I admit they are a dramatic and transparently defective lot but then so am I. They release me from the reality of the evening surgery. They have a certain style about them.

Katie suffers from another condition that I can't find in the book either. It's called chronic Pinot Noir. Actually it is not really chronic, it's intermittent acute Pinot Noir. I can tell when she's in an attack because her eyes take on a watery distant look. She also puts on more make-up than usual. I enjoy the way her lipstick never quite matches up to the contour of her lips. It either extends sideways up her cheek or wobbles along the top of her upper lip. The redness is in such contrast to her powder white face. She has certain priorities concerning this.

'If I die, Chris,' she once said, 'you will make sure I've got my lipstick on and my earrings in, won't you, dear?'

In an attack she talks in a confidentially refined voice that is filtered through gin and tonic. There's always a hint that we've known better days in which I am included as a confederate. We are both sophisticates that are temporarily slumming it. These indispositions graduate from gin into red wine evenings and then red wine days until I admit her to our cottage hospital to reduce the hues to a lighter shade.

Last time we did quite well for the first three days but on the fourth things started to slide away. I knew that smile with its slurred angle at the corner of the mouth and the gaze past my right ear. She was gently ticking.

Somewhere a bottle was hidden. I took on an un-accustomedly assertive role. I ransacked the room. I searched her case, her locker, under the bed, everywhere – nothing. I went into the bathroom. Perhaps she had. . . I lifted the lid of the lavatory cistern. There is was. An amphibious bottle of gin gently cooling in the stream. All it needed was some ice floating around and a sprig of mint on the ballcock – even perhaps some slices of lemon. You see, my advanced eccentrics have a certain style about them.

C. G. ELLIS
South Africa

Drug Smuggling

There are increasing reports of illicit drugs being smuggled through Customs using a variety of methods. Various techniques, including radiology and urine drug screening, have been reported to be useful in the detection of such smugglers.

A man in his 20's presented with clinical signs and symptoms suggestive of intestinal obstruction. Radiologically, this was confirmed as a small intestinal obstruction. He required surgery and at laparotomy the obstruction was at a Meckel's diverticulum where two fully-filled 'french letters' had impacted. It transpired that he had been in Morocco some three days previously where he had swallowed two 'french letters' stuffed with cannabis. Although there is controversy about methods of detection of drug smugglers with body packing, there was no doubt in this case. He was described as a genuine case of 'pot belly'.

AJIT SHAH
London

Custer's Last Stand

Members of the Flasher Fraternity vary as much in their size, shape, colour and creed as they do in the techniques they adopt. This could be prettily exemplified by the modus operandi of the accused which, if nothing else, had the virtue of originality. His tactic, apparently, was to pull his car into the kerb alongside his selected victim, roll down the window, smile politely as though about to ask directions, and then, when her attention was engaged, he would jerk his thumb in the direction of his exposed crotch.

How many successful forays our smiling cavalier had notched up only he alone knew. His last stand, however, was to be staged in the High Street of a Surrey dormitory town where the selected victim, a spinster of uncertain age, was, as events proved, not in the slightest degree amused by the encounter. Notwithstanding, she kept her cool, and noted down with admirable precision a description of the alleged culprit, the time and place of the alleged offence, together with details of the car and its registration number, all in all, sufficient for the police to proceed to a prosecution.

At the trial, the complainant proved to be an excellent witness who resolutely refused to be intimidated by the bully-boy tactics of defence counsel. At one juncture in the course of his abrasive cross-examination he paused, fiddled with the tail of his wig, pulled at the lapels of his well-worn gown, sure signs to the initiated that he was about to deliver what he obviously calculated would be a coup de grâce, 'Did he have an erection?', he brayed. 'No, sir,' she retorted calmly and unhesitatingly, 'He had a yellow Datsun.'

HENRY R. ROLLIN
Epsom

4 Psychoanalysis

A recording of Freud was the high spot of this year's annual general meeting of the Belsize Park Psychoanalytical Association. The gathering listened in dead silence, and you could cut the awe and reverence with a knife but, as the master spoke in German, nobody understood a word! They turned to an elderly German emigré and asked, 'What does he say?' He replied, 'Freud says the most important thing is to keep a kosher house.'

The Shrink

(after W. S. Gilbert)

I am the very model of a modern psychoanalyst,
I've got more clever answers than an 'Any Questions'
    panellist,
I've undergone analysis, both Freudian and Kleinian
And written up a thesis even though it's just a tiny 'un.
I've seen my training clients under guidance supervisory,
(The process is expensive, while the income is derisory)
I've studied learned volumes which were quite
    incomprehensible,
And sat in seminars which were comparatively sensible.
I've learned about the mental state of suffering humanity
From trivial neurosis to the borders of insanity;
My future publications, of which I intend to plan a list
Will prove that I'm the model of a modern psychoanalyst.

I recognize depression, both reactive and endogenous,
I've psycho-sexual skills for aberrations erotogenous,
I trifle with obesity and toy with anorexia,
Find fetishes are fun, but nymphomania is sexier.
I welcome the hysteric, the compulsive, the obsessional
In confidence as secret as the seal of the confessional,
Your complex I'll unravel, of Electra or of Oedipus,
And sort out your fixation on your mangy pup or seedy puss.
And if your symptom's not included in this miscellanea

No problem's so bizarre but I've encountered something
  zanier.
Of all the other ills I treat I'll gladly let you scan a list
To demonstrate my talents as a modern psychoanalyst.

In fact, when I can understand Jung's 'animus' and
  'anima',
Distinguish 'parent, adult, child' from grandpapa and
  granny-ma,
When I can hold a session without taking books by Freud
  with me
To quote them *in extenso* if the patient's paranoid with me,
When I can overcome my narcissistic insecurity
To practice my profession in its undiluted purity,
Can cope with countertransference, and fathom fact from
  fantasy,
You'll say of all the analysts in town I am the man to see.
In short, my erudition and consulting skills are laudable,
And though the clients may complain my fees are
  unaffordable,
They'll find a single consultation more convincing than a
  list
Of reasons why I am a model modern psychoanalyst.

MARIE CAMPKIN
London

Plus Ça Change, Plus C'est la Même Chose

John Eldon was an enthusiastic young doctor, having
passed through medical school with flying colours. He
decided his talents merited the strenuous tests of general
practice. By nature he disliked change, and wanted to settle
down in a community where he would be a pastor to his
flock. In this respect he resembled his 18th century ancestor,
Lord Eldon, who had maintained throughout the industrial
revolution that all change was for the worse. From these high

Tory origins, the genetic baton had been handed down to render him scornful of fashions in medicine. In his father's day there had been no nonsense. Then, the GP was a man of rugged individualism and undoubted authority who would dexterously evert the lower eyelid and declare to the patient: 'You're short of iron and anaemic' and then prescribe. No wonder he was a loved and respected figure in the neighbourhood. But how things have changed! Nowadays the GP is a more uncertain figure who seeks clues while he listens to and observes the patient who eventually tells him what is wrong!

In the old days there had been physical signs like rose spots or the mitral murmur, and methods like the coin test which made one certain of what one was dealing with. Now the trainer insisted that you kept a low profile to listen and observe. See him scratching the back of his head? That's self attack, due to confusion and mounting aggression. The next patient spoke with her hand across her mouth. She was a liar, and so on. It had always been the case. Nothing had changed about body language until Dr Morris wrote it up. It was not a fashion, like bad backs. In former times they were an affliction of aged gardeners: now, as his trainer pointed out, men in the middle 30s were chiefly affected. 'They work in offices by day, and watch television in the evening. The cause is undoubtedly due to *sex athletiformis*' said the trainer, who went on to deplore the change in sexual practice in his long spell as a GP. Dr Eldon liked his trainer, not only for his decisive pronouncements, but for that steady view of life that came from regular attendance at Church every Sunday.

By the end of his training, Dr Eldon felt ready to enter practice. He had been greatly interested in communication as the key to good practice. It was always stressed at group discussions with the course organizer. He identified himself most closely with his distant ancestor when communicating with old people. They were not verbose and spoke in condensed statements. They, like Lord Eldon, saw all change as being for the worse. They saw the odious winds of change blowing away old buildings, and streets full of memories. Fields were being devastated to make way for new office buildings, desirable apartments, drive-in supermarkets, and eight-lane motorways for commuter towns. When he said this was progress they told him he would change as he grew older. Perish the thought! One old man had gone as far as to say that a merciful Providence had allowed everything to deteriorate during a single life time to enable him to become reconciled with death! He did not have his hand across his mouth either. He went on, 'The summers have got worse, music louder and more senseless, the buildings uglier, the roads more congested, the trains slower and dirtier, governments sillier, and the news more depressing.' When Dr Eldon reported this case to the trainee group, they were united in the view that the old man was depressed and needed tricyclic antidepressants. Dr Eldon had his doubts. One of his main aims was to have a Porsche in the garage; not, as many thought to go careering about, because such a car would simply produce frustration when forced to drive at 15 mph, but to gloat over in much the same way as a Japanese banker gloats over a painting by van Gogh.

Being a good communicator, having a special interest in other people's emotional problems, presentable in appearance, and on the obstetric list, Dr Eldon soon found himself accepted in a three-man practice. It also helped that he read *The Times* and had a good public school background.

It was an outer-city practice consisting of many old residents living in run-down properties, a sizeable group of yuppies buying their first home, and a number of ethnic minority groups ensuring that the area was well supplied with Chinese, Tandoori and other restaurants supplying take-away Doner Kebabs. There were some local industries for the manufacture of foam cushions, furniture, toys and brush-making.

The partners – a male aged 68 and a female of 49, made him very welcome. Recognizing his interest in psychotherapy, they promised to refer him cases that would exploit his special skills. 'You don't need me to tell you that it's essential to preserve a sense of humour', said Dr Ross, the senior partner. 'We had to laugh the other day, Dr Lewis and I, when we encountered Mrs Bernstein in the corridor. She has always been a bit hypomanic and boastful. She asked after our families, and Dr Lewis said how proud she was of her 28 year-old son since he had just been made chief accountant of his company. She then turned to me and I told her that I had a grandson aged only 24 who had already become the managing director of his company. But, Mrs Bernstein was determined not to be outdone. 'I am delighted for both of you', she said 'but really that is nothing to compare with *my* grandson. He is only 18, but already he is helping the police with their enquiries!' Dr Eldon agreed that a GP must have a good sense of humour, and balancing outside interests. His own was cricket, at which he had performed very well at public school.

He was settling down in the practice when, a few weeks later, he received a letter from a local solicitor. It stated that he was representing a patient named Collymore (Winston) who had been convicted of assault and possessing a dangerous weapon, and needed a medical opinion on him. An appointment had been made for one morning next week. When the day came, Winston Collymore, an Afro-Caribbean patient originally from Barbados, entered with another young man from the same region, with his left arm in a sling, and heavily bandaged about the chest. 'I was only expecting one person,' began Dr Eldon. 'Oh! this is my friend, Silvester', said Winston, by way of introduction, 'He wanted to come with me'. 'I see,' said Dr Eldon, 'but what's happened to you?' 'He done it,' replied Silvester. 'We had an argument, and he stabbed me with a knife. I've had 27 stitches in my chest and arm.' 'But you're still friends?' asked Dr Eldon, somewhat flabbergasted. 'Sure, Doc, we're friends. We just had an argument.' 'But', said Dr Eldon, still confused, 'It must have been very serious!' 'Yes, it was, doc,' said Winston. 'What was it about?' asked Dr Eldon, 'a girl?' 'No, doc,' answered Silvester, laughing, 'It was much more serious than that. We was arguing about cricket!' At this, Dr Eldon gave way to emotion, and exclaimed 'Cricket? Why, that's a beautiful and peaceful game. I can't imagine anyone would get worked up to that extent over cricket.' At this, both Winston and Silvester stopped smiling and became serious as Winston raised his right index finger to make his point. 'Look, doc,' he said, 'You fight over football 'cos you takes it seriously. We takes cricket seriously. That's all.' Dr Eldon found this hard to answer, and even more difficult to explain in his letter to the solicitor.

More and more the vagaries of the human mind began to occupy Dr Eldon. He read widely, and probed more deeply. He became deeply interested in the work of Freud, the unconscious, and the interpretation of dreams. He now began to ask patients to whom he had listened to write down their dreams. This soon brought rewards, first of all in the case of Mr Sinclair, a 36 year-old civil servant, who had begun suffering from impotence. 'We have done all the physical tests, and can find nothing wrong, so we must turn our attention to those underlying forces which lurk hidden from our conscious experience. I should like you to record any dreams you have, to keep a pencil and paper by the bed, and report them to me.' It was not long before Mr Sinclair appeared, clutching a sheet of A4 on which were notes written with scrupulous, even obsessive care. This is the summary of what had been recorded:

I dreamed that I had died, and was standing in a short queue outside the pearly gates. It was all very different from what I had imagined because the recording angel wore a suit and stood before a kind of glass entrance, carrying a portable computer in his hand. He called the first man forward, and explained that judgement was made on the life below on one sin only, adultery. Depending on the record called up on the computer, one was provided with transport in accordance with the degree of adultery committed. At this, the man looked a bit edgy, while the angel operated the computer. Suddenly it began to emit buzzing noises and flashing lights of great intensity. 'Oh dear', said the angel, 'this is far from good. All I can offer you, I'm afraid, is a second-hand Volkswagen Beetle!' The man conceded that he must pay for the good time he had had on earth, and passed through the gateway. The second man was given the same explanation, but this time only one or two lights flashed, whereupon the angel declared this to be an average record, for which a suitable form of transport would be a Volvo 360. Apparently satisfied, the man entered his new existence. The third man, which whom I felt a strange affinity, almost as though he were my *Doppelgänger*, proudly stepped forward, head held high. 'I have no fear' he declared, 'about what you will find. I have led a blameless life.' 'Let us see, then,' said the recording angel, and to his great surprise the computer remained silent, even when given a sceptical shake. 'Fine!' said the angel. 'This is most unusual. Step forward' and as he said this he beckoned respectfully, whereupon a superb Rolls Royce slowly advanced and stopped. 'I think you will like this for it has every comfort, including a bar and television. For you, with your excellent record we offer you only the best. Are you happy with it?' The man sat down inside, and lowered the electric window, and said 'I couldn't be more happy. Thank you very much.' And he drove off. Now you know how it is in dreams, you move about in time and place, but it must have been a month or so later that I found myself back in the same place, watching what went on. I saw the recording angel at work with his computer, at the head of the queue, when suddenly he turned back and went back through the pearly gates. He had seen the Rolls approaching, but had noted that the driver did not look as happy as he should, so he waved him down. 'Is everything all right with the car?' he enquired. 'Oh, yes' came the answer. 'I stopped you because, from the look on your face, I felt you were not happy.' 'Well, you're quite right' said the driver, 'I'm not at all happy!' 'But why is that?' enquired the recording angel, who now was puzzled. 'I'll tell you why' came the answer – 'I've just overtaken my wife riding an old bike.'

Dr Eldon thought this an amusing story, but his duty was to keep a straight face, and interpret the dream in the light of his patient's impotence. 'I think I should like to see your wife, if that could be arranged' he said, tactfully, 'but at the moment, I wouldn't tell her anything about this dream. We'll keep that between ourselves for the present.'

Next day, Dr Ross 'phoned up on the intercom. 'I've got a middle-aged man I'd like you to see. He's rather depressed, and as we're sort of friends at the golf club, I think it would be better for this sort of thing if you'd see him. It would be awfully kind.' 'Very well, Dr Ross, do send him along, I've got a cancellation.' A few moments later, there was a quiet knock on the door, and in came Mr Burgess. 'Call me George,' he said. 'I'm a friend of the practice, and have known Dr Ross for years.' 'Well, George, Dr Ross did tell me you're feeling a bit down. Can you tell me why?' 'That's easy,' he said 'I got married to a very ugly woman.' 'Oh dear!' said Dr Eldon. 'I can understand how you feel. That's bad.' 'It is, doctor, but it's not all that bad, because at least she's very well-off.' 'Oh well,' said Dr Eldon, encouraged, 'that's not too bad then.' 'Oh yes it is,' came the reply 'because she's bloody mean.' 'Oh dear,' said Dr Eldon, looking for clues, 'that's terrible!' 'It's better than you think,' he said, 'because she's just bought us a large house costing £500,000.' 'Ah!' said Dr Eldon, 'at least you've got plenty of room to get away from her!' 'Yes,' said George, 'that's what I thought. But we'd only been in it a month when it was destroyed by fire, and the insurance cover had not been completed.' 'Oh my God!' said Dr Eldon, feeling the full force of George's reactive depression in a wave of empathy. 'Now I understand. That's terrible!' But, did he observe a slight brightening of the eyes, and a faint glimmer of a smile? There was a long pause, as George Burgess drew himself up to complete the discussion. 'Well, it wasn't too bad, doctor. You see, she was in it at the time!' He laughed uproariously, due to the relief of months of tension, and Dr Eldon realized his depression arose as the result of prolonged stress. 'Come and see me again next week George, or Dr Ross, if you prefer. Anyway, thank you for telling me all this.' George went off, apparently greatly relieved after such ventilation.

Dr Eldon admired his Jamaican patients' resistance to change and their continued adherence to inherited beliefs. He attributed a higher incidence of schizophrenia in this normally outgoing people to change of habitat. They showed little concern for the greenhouse effect, acid rain, or the ozone layer. They remained stable when steeped in their culture, like dear, fat Wilmer who, when Dr Eldon had admiringly pinched her baby's cheeks, scolded him by saying 'How you does be so wicked? You'll give the pickney a big ugly jaw. And now look at you, tickling her feet. Jesum piece! That'll give her a stutter and may even stop her talking!' Obviously, no one had ever tickled Wilmer's feet when she was a baby, but Dr Eldon recalled he had to be careful ever since that antenatal visit in June when he had advocated strawberries for their high vitamin C content, and Wilmer had remonstrated: 'Eat strawberries when you expecting, and pickney'll be born with a strawberry mark all over its poor face!' Best not to try and educate these patients, but leave them to such simple anxieties, for they're easier to avoid than atmospheric pollution. If success in psychiatry depends on change, it depends on a reversion to simpler elements.

Dr Eldon's interest in psychotherapy originated when he was at public school when for some reason they were asked to disclose the profession of their father. All went well at first as boys announced paternal origins such as clergyman, race-horse owner, or admiral. Then came poor Blowfield who, inhibited and stumbling, revealed that his school fees derived from the output of a toilet-roll factory, and thereafter became depressed and introverted. It would have been quite different had he been born in Japan! If only one could intervene to prevent the infliction of psychic damage in youth!

Then, one day, out of the blue such an opportunity seemed to present itself. At the end of morning surgery the 'phone went. It was the receptionist saying: 'Sorry to bother you at this time, Dr Eldon, but I've got an unusual problem. It concerns Miss Brenda White who's been brought in by her employer Mr Garson, the managing director of the local brush factory. He's not our patient, but he seems more upset and anxious than she is. I think I should explain that Brenda White is a poor 16 year-old who is a bit backward, but has been working at Brushes Ltd. for the past six weeks by arrangement with the Social Services Department to see how she gets on. Unfortunately, it seems, the women have to change into working overalls in a communal changing room where there is no privacy.' 'Yes, yes, Mrs Harper, please get to the point!' 'Well, doctor, it appears that Brenda is a late developer and is only just developing – you know – pubic hair, and the others have been teasing her that she's getting brush disease. Of course, it's gradually getting worse, and this morning she couldn't stand it any longer, and rushed up to Mr Garson's office saying she wanted to resign. So, he's brought her down for your professional authority to convince her that this is not a disease, but normal development, because she won't believe him.' 'I see,' said Dr Eldon. 'Thanks Mrs H., send them in.'

A few moments later, Brenda was brought in by Mr Garson, who did indeed appear much the more nervous of the two. Dr Eldon stood up and shook him firmly by the hand, saying 'It's all right, I think I know what's brought you along. Sit down Brenda.'

'Well, doctor, ' began Mr Garson, 'I don't think it's going to be all that simple, even for you. Could we just have a word in private?'

'Why yes, excuse us just a minute, Brenda. I'll get you a magazine to look at.' Dr Eldon then led Mr Garson into his side room and said, reassuringly, 'Don't worry, we'll soon sort this out.' Mr Garson sat down, and resumed his managerial demeanour. 'I wouldn't be too certain about that, Dr Eldon. You've only been told part of the story. You see, she came rushing into my office this morning, blurting out this rubbish about brush disease. I explained patiently that this was a very healthy industry, but she refused to believe me. So I asked her what form it took, and when she explained, I had to laugh and tell her this was something quite normal that happened to us all as we grew up. Then it was that I made my big mistake! Seeing I could not persuade her, I got up from my desk and went over and locked the door. The only way to convince her would be to show myself to her to explain that pubic hair was natural and that we were all the same. So I came back into the room, lowered my trousers and pulled up my shirt and said 'There you are, Brenda, look at me. . . But, before I could say another word she had jumped to her feet shrieking: 'Oh, Gawd, Sir! Ain't you got it bad – you've got the 'andle 'n all!!!' It was then Dr Eldon had to admit his first professional defeat.

M. KEITH THOMPSON
Croydon

Baby Talk

I love my mum, I love my dad
And I am quite contented
I wish old nutty Sigmund Freud
Had never been invented.

Clerihew

Psychiatrists are full of its and buts,
And mostly they are clearly nuts.

Life's Work

Dreams of Id and Super-Ego
Potty training, self-abuse
Filled young Sigmund's every moment
Though none of it was any use.

Oedipus Complex

Siggy's mum loved Siggy's tum,
Siggy loved her breast.
This complicated love-life
Made everyone depressed.

Siggy's dad said it was bad
And bought the boy a dummy
But he had read of Oedipus
and how HE loved his mummy.

Siggy's thoughts about the sports
He fancied with his mother
Started psychoanalysis
And caused a lot of bother.

Grilled Soul

I am a Freud, Ian, you are too Jung
To enter the profession.
What do you know of Mother Love,
Of Anal Fixed Aggression?

How do you handle breasts, my boy,
And is your Id a yob?
Get out and get Analysis
Better still, a proper job.

RICHARD WYNDHAM
Marlingford

5 Psychogeriatrics

*T*his is an umbrella title* covering both elderly doctors and elderly patients. If you aspire to the image of scientist, elder statesman, philosopher, it is essential to learn half a dozen easy quotations from Popper (Teilhard de Chardin is even better) and apply them indiscriminately to any problem situation – as Popper calls it – or just problem, as we say in Twickenham. As Popper puts it, 'It is impossible to speak in such a way that you cannot be misunderstood'; so don't fight it, utter delphically, and you will soon be asked to do the Harveian Lecture at the Royal College of Physicians. David Pyke, of that College, quotes Medawar (not bad) to the effect that ageing is a funny thing. When Sir Peter first had to get reading glasses, he said 'Now I know what those little furry things are I work with. They're mice.'

Blodwen and the Cause of It All

'Watsacausathatthen, Doctor?'

Most of the patients that I met in my trainee year 'talked Swansea', but none were a patch on Blodwen Davies. I'd see her at the surgery at least once a week, and always it would be the same. She wouldn't wait for me to call her name but would bolt for my door as soon as the previous patient exited. Then, no time to draw breath, a long list of symptoms, usually intestinal with a smattering of psychosis, followed by the inevitable coda; 'Watsacausathatthen, Doctor?' Of course I never, ever knew, but she seemed happy enough with my vague mumblings and the occasional prescription for Mist. Mag. Trisil.

---

*'What did Queen Victoria say when she came to the throne?' 'I think I'm going to reign.'

Years ago, my training practice had nestled deep in the heart of some of the worst slums in South Wales. The little two-up two-down terraces had marched up the hillside overlooking the bay. Their tightly-packed, back-to-back ranks had, despite their proximity to the docks, survived the worst of Swansea's blitz. Then 20 years on, they met their match, the City Council Planning Department. The Victorian terraces were demolished and a criss-cross swathe of dual carriage way was laid upon the area like some giant cross.

All the inhabitants were rehoused of course. This being the 1960s and there not being quite as much space as there had been, due to half the area being under tarmac, high-rise had to be the answer. And so, in the arms of the cross, Swansea Council created Dafaty Flats, a sort of purgatory in the vertical.

Blodwen lived half-way up the southernmost tower block, and our practice occupied a dingy health centre two miles away on the northern edge of the bitumen desert. However, for as long as any of the receptionists could remember, this 73 year-old spinster had dragged herself up to one of our surgeries on at least a weekly basis. As is traditional with such patients, she had long ceased to be seen by anyone but the trainee. 'A good example of the limitations of primary care' was how my trainer used to describe her, and his eyes would glaze over as I reported on her latest symptoms. After all what could anyone do? One would have to be incurably insane, or demented, or both, to do what Blodwen did each week. The eight snarling lanes of 'urban freeway' traffic that she had to negotiate were not to be faced lightly at the best of times, and, come rain or shine, she always walked to the surgery. Mad.

Then, one day, something amazing happened, Blowden asked for a house-call. I should have realized that something was up; it had been nearly a fortnight since her last appointment.

I drew to a halt beneath Blodwen's flat. I was lucky. The council, in their infinite wisdom, had provided spaces for ten cars per block of 50 flats. I suppose the rationale was that anyone poor enough to have to carry on living in Dafaty Flats was too poor to run a car. Of course, they were absolutely right, but that did not stop people from trying to anyway.

I managed to squeeze in between an old Cortina with four flat tyres and a burnt out rusty heap that vaguely resembled a Morris Marina. Its tyres may have been fine; it was difficult to tell — it had no wheels.

I had had a lot of experience of home visits at Dafaty flats. Perhaps the partners thought that my car blended into the local scenery better than their newer models. I had discovered that an immutable law applied to home visits there. I was proud of this law, which I felt sure must be universal. I called it Jones' law; the likelihood of the lift working is inversely proportional to the height above ground of your patient.

Blodwen lived on the eighth floor. It was a long climb. At least the grafitti were interesting. Gasping for breath, I pressed the door bell of Number 87. From somewhere deep within, a ghastly, muted, electronic warble played 'We'll Keep a Welcome in the Hillside.' Preceded by much shuffling and muttering, Blodwen opened the door. 'Ooh! Doctor! Good of you to come.'

As I stood there, I noticed the first unusual thing about Number 87. All the stairwells in the blocks had their own powerful odour, a heady cocktail of vomit, stale alcohol and excrement, all laced with a powerful disinfectant. Blodwen's flat was unique in my experience; it actually smelt worse. She ushered me into her tiny living room and I noticed something else rather odd. There, lined up neatly on the mantelpiece, were at least two dozen brown medicine bottles. I inspected Blodwen's strange ornaments.

Working my way along the row I realized that they were bottles of Mist. Nag. Trisil., each one dustier and older than the last. Halfway along, the labels changed; it seemed that my predecessor had favoured 'Gaviscon'. Nearly all the bottles were full. Blodwen looked faintly embarrassed. 'Well, I tries 'em sometimes, but they don't seem to do much. An' I know you've got to learn your doctoring somewhere. I didn't want to dishearten you like.'

She quickly moved on to describe her symptoms. They seemed much the same as ever, only worse. But this time there was one important difference, she really did look ill. Her eyes were sunken and she was whiter than any sheet in

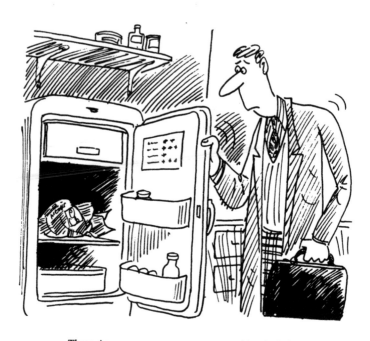

There, in some greasy newspaper, something lurked.

the place. Poor Blodwen had to interrupt her tale to retch into the old washing-up bowl by her side.

'Could it have been anything you've eaten, do you think?' 'Scuse me, Doctor. No, I've had nothing unusual, just me normal bit o' pork from the market. . .' She broke off and dived for the bowl once more.

I wandered into the kitchen, I thought she could do with a sip of water. If anything the kitchen smelled worse than the living room. Scraps of mouldy food lay on every surface. I felt that I might catch something just by inhaling too deeply. As I filled the least dirty mug I could find, I noticed the fridge next to the sink. Its door was ajar. I peered into its murky, and obviously unrefrigerated, depths. There, in some greasy newspaper, something lurked.

'Err, Blodwen, What's in the fridge?' 'That's me bit o' pork, love. But don' worry. Mr Williams keeps that by special for me. Knows I can't afford nothing dear, so its two pound of belly pork. Regular, nice an' fresh. First Wednesday, every month.' My stomach was doing strange things beneath my rib cage. 'But, but today's the twenty-seventh.' 'Well, I've

I got to make my pension last. An' I keeps it in the fridge.'

As I examined her I gently explained that her fridge was not working, and that she really needed to give her tummy a rest for a while. Apart from a complete absence of any sense of smell, and a nasty case of gastroenteritis, I could find little seriously wrong with my patient. I advised sips of clear fluid only, and gave her an injection for the nausea. Before I left I held my breath and quickly stuffed the rancid belly pork into the bin. Blodwen seemed rather put out, but she cheered up when I promised to return the following day to see how she was getting along. I did want to review her, but I had also had an idea.

The following day Blodwen looked much better. I said that I had a surprise for her and disappeared into the kitchen. A few minutes work with a screw-driver, a new 13 amp fuse, and, rather to my surprise, the old lady's ancient refrigerator hummed into life once more. We had a long discussion about the merits of Mr Williams' best pork belly cuts and both agreed that one pound every fortnight would be a more sensible order. Pressing home my advantage, I asked her if she had ever thought of having meals-on-wheels or home help, She seemed rather keen on the idea.

As I manoeuvred out of the flats' car park I could not help feeling rather pleased with myself. A classic case of useful intervention in primary care, I reflected proudly, as I weaved a careful route between the smashed cider bottles and abandoned supermarket trolleys.

It really made my week, thinking about Blodwen. Who knows how long her fridge had been on the blink? That poor old duck had probably had chronic food-poisoning for ages and, just because she was a bit odd, no one had picked it up. She had been doomed to return to the health centre week after week, where, because we had all pigeon-holed her as 'daft', nobody listened to her any more. I sailed through my surgeries over the next few days. I didn't care how many sore throats or snotty noses I saw. After all, I was the trainee who had sorted out Blodwen Davies. My elation lasted until one moment after the third patient of my Friday afternoon surgery had left the room. A formidable, familiar shape filled the doorway.

'Ooh, 'ello Doctor. Sorry to bother you again, but. . .'

It was all new, I will give her that. Gone was the nausea and the wind and the tummy cramps. All swept away in an avalanche of new symptoms. Shooting pains in the legs; spots before the eyes; funny noises in the chest; and all of them 'chronic' or 'terrible' or 'diabolical'. She paused for breath, and then: 'Watsacausathatthen, Doctor?'

And so it went on. For my two remaining months with the practice, I saw Blodwen at least once a week. I never did sort out any of her new problems and, all too soon, it was time to hand over to the new trainee.

She seemed a nice girl. Keen. Reminded me of how I had felt when I arrived at the health centre. Together we went through the list of regular patients that she would be inheriting. We came to Blodwen Davies' name. 'Ah,' I paused, and my eyes swam out of focus as I gazed out of the grimy window. 'I expect you'll see a lot of her. A good example of the limitations of primary care.'

GERAINT JONES
Leiston

No Room at the Hostel

They used to be called 'Old Homes' but, just as the residents became transformed from pensioners to senior citizens, the bricks and mortar became changed into Homes for the Elderly and eventually, with the trend to computerization, we now have 'Part Three Hostels'. Although there is no official age limit for entry and, theoretically, one could take up residence at 16 years of age, straight from school – in practice, most of the residents are elderly and many are over 75 and still going strong.

Modern medicine has a lot to answer for, but the greatest sin by far is abolishing those killer diseases, like consumption and infantile paralysis, that used to prevent people earning their rightful place in the Part Three Hostel. Even at such advanced ages as 80 and 90, it is almost impossible to depart the earth, as relatives and keen health workers battle to save lives.

The concept of preserving mummified geriatrics in suspended animation for evermore is indeed laudible – after all the alchemists of old, when they were not trying to transmute base metals into gold, were also hankering after eternal life. The problem is that the care assistants entrusted with this lofty task do not appear to have read all the rules. It seems that inmates are welcome as long as they do not cause inconvenience. Inconvenience can be classified according to degree and person inconvenienced. Thus, environmental desecration, such as smearing excreta on walls, or piddling in potted plants, uttering foul language or stripping off in full view of other residents incurs maximum penalty points. Not far behind is social abuse, such as making procreative suggestions, or even attempting to mount residents, trying to escape, using violence when being assisted to dress, or simply adopting an aggressive attitude to fellow residents.

The other cardinal sin concerns the effect of these senile delinquent acts on the supervisors. Staff can be provoked into abject terror, threat of resignation or even strike unless 'something is done'. Of course, the only thing that must be done is to cast away the offender to an asylum where 'treatment' can be given. Unfortunately, even after the 'treatment', the inmate is not accepted back at the hostel, because the other inmates and the staff are too traumatized by the whole incident to take any further risks.

Maybe we can formulate an eleventh commandment: 'When thou shalt tend towards ageing, desist from abusing either thy fellow man or thine abode, or else thy keeper may yield unto temptation and cast thee out into oblivion.'

M.A. LAUNER
Burnley

Florence

Florence (Flo) was a large, loud lady with big bosoms, dirty straggling hair, and a dangling cigarette. She loved to reminisce about her days with the wartime concert party; and thumped out the good old tunes on the piano. Her mood disorder began when she was 33, with 15 subsequent admissions to hospital. Between episodes, only alcohol soothed her erratic moods.

Flo lived with her husband, Wayne, and their two ancient cats, Rusty and Felix. Unfortunately, when Flo was 75, Wayne and the cats all died. She was bereft and drank more. It so happened that Nick, a young man of Latin descent, who specialized in reading the obituary columns, was at hand. He contacted the widow to offer his services as a handyman. In her plight, she learned to lean on him, and in no time, he was fixing her house, having full use of her car, as well as her unquestioning love. As a token, she allowed him to mortgage her house for payment of services. At this point, however, her illness undid her and she was admitted to hospital.

Flo responded to treatment, but was found to be financially incompetent. She remained infatuated with Nick, and upon dischange, went to live with him and his wife. During this time, Nick tried hard to have the incompetency lifted, but the strain told and, being so worried about Flo's financial state, he had a row with his wife and hit her for the first time. This certainly upset Flo, but the final straw concerning readmission, was when she became confused and defaecated on the floor.

Flo again improved, but things began to unravel for Nick. The psychiatrist, doing a routine consultation at a nearby nursing home, encountered another old lady who knew Nick. She was now in straightened circumstances because she had given him the deeds of her house. Nevertheless, she still loved him and kept his picture close by. This was borrowed to show Flo, who duly recognized and gushed over it. The police were notified, and a Staff Sergeant came to sort things out. It turned out that caring for old ladies was Nick's occupation when he was not doing time. Notwithstanding being in bad odour with the police and the Public Trustee, Nick continued to profess concern for Flo's financial welfare until banned from the hospital. Flo thought it would be nice for Nick to be the executor of her will.

The denouement eventually came, and Nick had his day in court. The psychiatrist had carefully documented all the evidence, and expressed his deep concern about elder abuse. Lifting his eyes from his prepared text, he could see Flo gazing adoringly at Nick and blowing him kisses across the courtroom.

Nick got three years for fraud. Flo? She lives in a nursing home, exuberant as ever dribbling cigarette ash everywhere, and wondering about Nick.

W.C.M. SCOTT
Quebec, Canada

6 Child Psychiatry

A few weeks ago, I had to go to Glasgow to examine. I asked this youth, 'What is the cause of Down's syndrome'. He answered, 'In Scotland, the commonest cause of Down's syndrome is trisodomy 21' – hence, the expression, the Gay Gordons.

Such problems are common to all races, societies and creeds. When Chairman Hu succeeded Chairman Mao, the BBC announcer said that Hu is a friend of Dung Hsiao Ping and, like Dung, was purged during the Cultural Revolution. In this connection, a French colleague sent his son to us for a few weeks to learn English. On a return visit, we knocked at their door in Paris and the child opened it. 'Is your father at home?' I asked in that clear ringing tone one reserves for foreigners. 'Yes, he is,' he replied, 'He is doing No. 3.' Later, I reported this back to his father and added, 'The mind boggles.' 'Yes,' he said 'that is No. 3.'

Shrinking in the Large

Murphy's Law, as applied to psychiatrists encountering their clients in public, would say: such meetings in the main occur in circumstances that cause maximum embarrassment and discomfort to the psychiatrist.

It was thus, on a Saturday morning in Sainsbury's, not long after I had left London to take up my appointment as a consultant child psychiatrist in a provincial town, that I came to learn the real meaning of the term 'shrink'. I was doing the shopping, accompanied by my toddler daughter. Whilst we were searching a low shelf for the right brand of cereal, I was startled to hear my professional name called by a child some way off. Now doctors are used to hallucinating their name being called in public, diving towards 'phones that are either silent or ringing for someone else, but this was real. Looking up I was horrified to see hurtling towards us two shopping trolleys laden and surrounded by savage children waving and calling my name. Their haggard and preoccupied parents followed but appeared not yet to have seen me. I recognized them as a particularly demanding problem family that was seeing me in my Clinic for therapy. One of their wild children pointed at me and shouted 'shrink!'. I did just that, diving behind the nearest counter which happened to be pet food, coming face to face with a bag of 'Winalot'. I am about to lose a lot, I thought ironically, remembering how much of my time the family would demand if they managed to corner me. In fact the way therapy was going they would undoubtedly make me feel like a dartboard. I bent low and managed to escape further recognition but in the process let go of my active daughter who rushed forward to greet the entourage, blocking its progress. To my embarrassment I overheard the 'problem' parents sternly exclaim: 'Why can't some people look after their kids!' as they plucked my daughter from their path and rushed her as lost to the nearest check-out point. Moments later I sheepishly reclaimed her from the cashier, a teenage girl who also, regrettably, looked professionally familiar.

As if this was not enough, I failed to shrink successfully in a furniture shop a week later. This time I was actually collared by, believe it or not, the same family. They were in a state of crisis and demanded an on-the-spot consultation. 'Do these things only happen me?' I wondered all the way home, only to find that in my distraction following the meeting, I had purchased the very lamp in the sale my wife had *not* set her heart on. 'Never mind, dear,' I said 'As it's late I'll 'phone the shop straight away and reserve the right one before it goes'. Still preoccupied by my encounter I took the receipt from the purchase I had made and dialled the shop's number several times, only to be further distressed by each time receiving on the other end someone speaking an unintelligible foreign language. My wife came to the rescue: 'What on earth's wrong with you? You're dialling their VAT number!' she explained, pointing out the shop's proper 'phone number on the receipt. Such is the traumatic nature of such encounters, at least on the psychiatrist.

Further unplanned and sometimes embarrassing 'shrinking' encounters with clients in public seemed to follow with

alarming frequency. I began suffering nightmares – in one I
was trapped in a lift with a problem family I was treating,
whose children were eating ice-creams. My daughter,
beyond my control, snatched the other children's ice-creams
and proceeded to ram them into their faces. In another, I
dreamt I was conducting my clinic in my pyjamas with
everyone around me, in true British style, too polite to
comment. In waking life, whenever I ventured out in public,
I began to imagine clients everywhere – in front, to the side,
and especially behind me, undoubtedly scrutinizing my
relationships with my own family. Were clients singling me
out? I even saw in a new light the behaviour of an ex-client,
a paranoid psychotic, who suffered similar feelings. When
out in the street he had worn around his head a band with
car wing mirrors protruding on either side so as to see behind
him. At this early stage in my career I was too embarrassed
to confess my experiences to my senior colleagues. It can be
lonely being a psychiatrist – I even fleetingly thought of
writing (anonymously, of course) to one of the agony aunts.
At length, though, I began looking at the situation rationally
– meeting clients in public, outside the snug formality of the
professional relationship in the clinic, was something I was
unprepared for, having been thoroughly spoilt by the
anonymity of London. I had never seemed to need to 'shrink'
there. I was, of course, in my provincial practice undergoing
the process I now understand of 'becoming known.'
Perhaps, I reflected, one should just greet clients naturally –
though one would risk either demands for on-the-spot taxing consultations or their embarrassment ('this is my
psychiatrist', I could just hear one of them introducing me to
their friend. It would go down all right in America, but not
yet in Britain.) Yet to ignore each other would somehow
devalue the particularly intimate although stigmatized
relationship a psychiatrist, in contrast to other specialists, has
with his or her clients and lead to feelings of rejection. I say
'each other' implying the singular – of course the unease for
a modern child psychiatrist like myself, treating whole
families, is frequently multiplied by four or more.
   A dinner party with colleagues not long afterwards
confirmed I was not alone in suffering unfortunate
encounters with clients and the general public. I was thus

prompted to begin my research into their nature and
phenomenology. At the party, after sufficient ethanolic
priming, the confessions began to flow. The 'winner' that
evening must surely have been Dr A who described an
experience as a psychiatric trainee fresh from a politically
unstable country where terrorism was rife. She had left her
briefcase in her car in a notoriously villain-infested car park
whilst attending a lecture at the district general hospital. On
return, whilst driving 'home' (the psychiatric hospital in
which she was a resident) she heard a ticking coming from
her case. She became increasingly concerned that a time-
bomb had been planted, so much so that on arrival at the
psychiatric hospital she immediately 'phoned the police.
Moments later several squad cars, including a bomb disposal
unit from the local army headquarters, sirened to halt and
cordoned off the area of her car. In front of a large audience
of psychiatric patients that had by now gathered, the bomb
disposal experts delicately extracted the brief case and blew
it open. Amongst the debris they found the cause of the
sinister noise – in her case she had left her pocket
Dictaphone switched on and it had run out of tape. In front
of the amused crowd, really wishing to shrink, she quietly
apologized to the experts. 'Not at all,' they said, 'we must
thank you. We are always looking for opportunities to
practice'. At the dinner party, Dr A dryly added 'The event
left its impact on my patients – I know I subsequently starred
in several delusions as a terrorist spy'.

Several weeks later, as Christmas approached, I was in my
clinic changing into a rather tight-fitting Cub-Scout uniform,
reflecting that at least one is safe from unsolicited encounters
in one's own clinic. I was also churning over the problems
of trying to research 'shrinking' – my experience so far
suggested the normal controls would certainly perform
better than the subject group of psychiatrists. Also, need
impromptu encounters with one's clients be traumatic? If so,
for whom? Perhaps clients benefit from seeing us as human
and fallible. Oh, about the Cub uniform – I was about to
leave my clinic to attend a paediatric department fancy dress
lunch – not that in my present state of near bursting I would
risk eating much. As I opened the door of my office and
entered the corridor my Cub cap fell off. I stooped to pick it

up as just opposite the door of my social worker colleague's office opened . . . she later described the incident thus: 'I was preparing a rather nervous family to meet Dr – at their next appointment. The family had reservations about psychiatrists based on unsuccessful treatment from one they described as 'bizarre' in the past. 'Dr – is quite different. He's very up to date and at the same time down to earth. You'll meet him soon.' I reassured the family as I was showing them out of my office 'Oh, there is Dr – . . .'. I had already blurted out his name when the family and myself froze as we saw in front of us an over-sized Cub-Scout in full uniform, adjusting his cap. An implement knife dangled nonchalantly from his belt'. Thus an addendum to Murphy's Law is that a psychiatrist must not regard himself as immune from the need to shrink in his or her clinic either.

'A psychiatrist is basically appointed by a Health Authority to enhance the normality of his region,' I could imagine the GMC saying, 'therefore for one to behave in abnormal or indiscreet ways in public . . .' Of course that's a major problem! My research was beginning to show that it is precisely the desire of young psychiatrists to retain their own normality which prompts them to take drastic (often panic) measures to extricate themselves from embarrassing situations. It is these measures, though, which so often make the original problem so much worse. This is illustrated by the case of Dr B who, freshly appointed from the capital, was enthusiastic to introduce family therapy to the shires. He was about to give a role play demonstration of a family therapy session to an audience of Health Visitors gathered in his Clinic. Of an inventive nature, Dr B had brought a large teddy bear to play the part of the baby in the family session that was otherwise to be acted by his colleagues and himself. En route from his car to the clinic he carried the bear across a shopping precinct. As he did so, the smiling faces around him led him to reflect pleasantly on the friendliness of his new home town. Suddenly Dr B realized the faces belonged to a large family he was treating. When he grasped that the teenage children were pointing and giggling at the teddy bear he tried to hide it under his coat. So far, so good. But he lost his grip on the bear, which slithered to the ground. Poor Dr B! If only he had shown the poise to have asked one of the youngsters to pick it up for him. Instead, the portly Dr B stooped to retrieve his large furry actor. He said at the 'post mortem' later: 'I experienced a ripping sound followed by a cold air blast from behind which struck at the part of my anatomy that indicated the tear in my trousers had occurred in a fatal region.' Seeking refuge in an adjacent hardware shop, he purchased a tube of Bostik glue which he used to effect a desperate and temporary repair. Imagination suggests how, not long afterwards, this attempted solution proved more painful than the original embarrassment. The incident heralded a permanent aversion to bending which, with Dr B's encouragement, many confused with sciatica.

The above case history from my research illustrates another point: the techniques of modern family therapy can create difficulties for the inexperienced child and adolescent psychiatrist aspiring to normality. This was brought home to me whilst doing a domiciliary visit on a warm, gentle family allowing themselves to be terrorized by a 'monster' teenage son. The parents plied me with coffee while their son refused to partake in the session, having locked himself in his room, I began to feel quite stuck as to how to intervene. Looking out of the french windows at their lovely garden I decided to take a break. Now this is something psychiatrists using family therapy frequently do when stuck – it merely means extricating onself (either alone or with one's co-worker) from the family for a short while to reflect on what is happening and to plan a strategy before returning. So I said to the family 'I would like to take a break for a few moments.' The kindly mother rushed forward to show me the toilet. 'It's all right, thank you,' I said, 'I prefer to go to the bottom of your garden'. The parents looked at each other, shocked. Standing in front of their rose-bed, contemplating their predicament, I was dimly aware of the parents, despite my having proffered further explanation, still glancing at me anxiously.

A consistent finding in my research, though, is that there is always a better story to be found. During a discussion on the contribution of having one's remarks misinterpreted in the aetiology of shrinking, Dr C, an adult psychiatrist, told me about an incident when he was invited to lecture on marital and sexual problems to a local mental health support group containing many ex-clients. He had a few slides of graphs to show and his projectionist was a strikingly attractive young lady. When Dr C had finished showing his slides and no longer wanted the projector on he shouted across the hall to the projectionist. 'Can we have it off, please?'

So far my research has highlighted the problems of younger, less experienced psychiatrists. Have older colleagues managed to find ways to escape ordeal with embarrassing encounters? Alas, not entirely. As age advances the problems of memory can strike anywhere and knock the normality out of even the most distinguished psychiatrist. After a while everyone in a provincial town comes to look vaguely familiar without being sufficiently specifically so. Many are ex-clients. But just because someone looks unfamiliar does not mean you are safe, as a provincially installed bachelor psychiatrist colleague pointed out. He was attempting familiarity with a beautiful young lady at a party and began with the cliche (fatal to psychiatrists) 'Haven't I seen you somewhere before?', to which she replied 'Yes, I was your patient before you cured me of anorexia!'

Unfortunately, the situation arrives all too soon where one's memory play tricks with current clients. A busy senior family psychiatrist rushed to collect her next appointment from the crowded waiting room. Ushering a large family into her office she reflected, in current family therapy style, 'Good, they've brought their relatives too.' As the session began she was struck by the lack of communication between various portions of the family. 'Interesting,' she thought, 'This explains why some of the children are showing symptoms.' It was only when she confronted the family with their communication difficulties that the unfortunate psychiatrist discovered that, in her haste, she had shepherded into her room two unrelated families who had been waiting simultaneously for appointments with different practitioners in the clinic.

The winner in the 'more experienced' psychiatrist section must be Dr D who described his memory defect thus: 'One of my cerebral hemispheres remembers faces, the other names, but there are no connecting fibres.' He illustrated this with an incident in a train where he was sitting opposite a man, sternly reading his newspaper, who looked very familiar. Dr D's brain was tormenting him. Was this an ex-client. No, Dr D thought, he somehow looked too important. Worse, was he an old colleague that Dr D should acknow-ledge? The other man was too absorbed in reading to make eye contact. Dr D strained to activate his memory circuits. At last his other hemisphere came into play and supplied a name – the other man must surely have been a fellow resident psychiatric trainee in the distant past. Suddenly pleased with the return of his mental powers, Dr D used the greeting (pioneered between Freud and Jung) that had been so fashionable in his particular training group: 'You're all right; how am I?' The other man looked up astonished. Dr D realized he had got it wrong and began to apologize: 'It's just that you look awfully familiar!' 'I'm Michael Heseltine,' the other man retorted and immediately resumed his self-important stance behind his newspaper.

During my research I posed the question: 'Is meeting ex-clients in public easier if one has successfully treated them and the relationship has ended on a good note?' A fellow psychiatrist dashed this vain hope. He related an incident whereby upon returning to the road where he had parked his car he witnessed a traffic warden confidently delivering parking tickets to the entire row of cars while a queue of drivers angrily protested. As she slapped one on the psychiatrist's car, he recognized her as a lady he had treated (unfortunately with success) for social phobia and lack of assertiveness. As the psychiatrist lamented to me: 'My own assertiveness on this occasion did not lead to a modification of her behaviour.'

As yet, there are no recommendations from the Royal College of Psychiatrists on how to handle impromptu 'shrinking' encounters between psychiatrists and their clients. Nor is the matter tackled in training. For this reason a colleague is preparing a practical handbook on the subject entitled *Tricks for Psychlists*. In considering the uncomplicated 'brush against' shopping-type encounter which may be embarrassing to clients, she advocates the psychiatrist's use of the perfunctory ambiguous nod, a mild greeting barely discernible to most unless they are looking for it. Such a nod leaves the initiative for any further social intercourse to the

client (who is also entitled to shrink). However, it can
sometimes be confused as a tic, especially when used
continuously by the well-established psychiatrist who is
beginning to experience eveyone looking familiar. She
suggests that the nod (in pre-tic moderation) could be
cultivated in psychiatric trainees by the simple use of a
mirror. If clients attempt to load you with their problems in
public the guide recommends advising them, gently but
firmly, that they need to find someone to talk to. The
handbook also recommends various preventive measures to
reduce the need for shrinking, including avoiding lifts,
elderly trousers, Butlins, video shops and taking toddlers
shopping.

Apart from meeting clients, shrinking can also occur when
out socially, someone discovers you are a psychiatrist and
you face being bombarded by tiresome personal revelations,
or, sometimes, rebuffs, especially if people fear you can X-ray
their minds. *Tricks for Psychlists* suggests employing various
euphemisms for our trade, including 'public relations,'
'personnel' and even 'psychological engineering' in order to
escape recognition. One psychatrist, though, decided to be
more original when he fancied a single lady at a party. By
telling her that he worked for the Electricity Board (in a sense
this was true as he had a particular interest in electro-
convulsive therapy), he hoped this would sound sufficiently
boring to steer the conversation away from his work and
towards more promising areas. However, the lady glowered
at him: 'You work for the Electricity Board? I've been trying
for three weeks to get you wretched people to come and
mend my cooker. . .' The strength of this tirade was matched
by the practitioner's regret at his little deceit.

An observation stands out from my research: very seldom
does one see one's very experienced much older psychiatric
colleagues out and about in public. Certainly, they avoid
shopping centres. I now know why – having suffered many
'shrinking' incidents, they have developed agoraphobia. The
truth is agoraphobia is more prevalent in psychiatrists than in
their clients. Withdrawing from social outings, particularly
shopping, may lead to stress in the marriage as spouses
often doubt the authenticity of the condition and suspect mal-
ingering. Thus, compensatory measures are necessary: one

colleague was pressurized by his wife into taking up DIY ('if you are going to sit at home all day long'). Rather than face such a grim prospect, this colleague developed an unprecedented interest in reading and research. As he put it 'a whole year's journals came out of their cellophane wrappers for the first time.' Where treatment is desired, whilst administering psychotherapy to patients, a psychiatrist may improve in his or her self-confidence and feel more able to face (and even turn to advantage) seeing his or her clients in public. Such effects may generalize. However, there is no research investigating to what extent psychiatrists themselves are helped by their treatments and the old adage that they are in their trade to cure themselves has never been put to the test.

Many psychiatrists, though, settle to benefit from their agoraphobia and move to the countryside a good distance from their workplace where they establish self-sufficient smallholdings (almost republics) that obviate the need to enter into public places such as shops. They just about manage to go to work and, perhaps, the golf course. In a few psychiatrists the condition worsens to the point where they increasingly look for opportunities to avoid seeing clients at all and instead take up more and more committee work. I suppose this is what is meant when they are described as a 'successful shrink'.

PETER J. HARDWICK
Poole

Better Late than Never

Shrink: Come in and sit down – uh – it's Andrew I believe?
Boy   : Andy.
Shrink: You prefer Andy to Andrew?
Boy   : That's right.
Shrink: Would it bother you if I called you Andrew?
Boy   : Suit yourself. What's your name?
Shrink: Dr Colder, but you can call me Frank if you want.
Boy   : 'Colder' is a funny name.
Shrink: Why do you say that?
Boy   : I don't know, it just sounds funny to me.

Shrink: Do you know why I've been asked to see you?

Boy   : Suppose you tell me; I bet you can guess what I'm thinking anyway.

Shrink: I'd rather you'd try and tell me yourself. It's you who's got to do most of the talking during our sessions together.

Boy   : What about?

Shrink: The things that bother you.

Boy   : What things?

Shrink: Well, you must be worried about something?

Boy   : Come off it!

Shrink: Perhaps you'd rather not talk about it?

Boy   : Are you really a doctor? You sure don't look like one.

Shrink: Yes, I am a doctor but probably not the sort you've come across before. I try and help people with their problems.

Boy   : What problems?

Shrink: Well, you might say problems in living.

Boy   : You mean nutter cases like Mr Thompson next door to us, who keeps talking to God.

Shrink: (Laughs) Not exactly, but it wouldn't be proper for me to discuss another doctor's case with you.

Boy   : I spoke to God once.

Shrink: Really?

Boy   : Yeah, I once asked him to send me a 10 gear bike for my birthday, but I only got a 5 gear one, so I gave him up as a bad job. It didn't even have a light.

Shrink: Wasn't that a bit hard on poor old God?

Boy   : All my mates got 10 gear ones with back and front lights.

Shrink: Do you think it's right to judge God or anyone else for that matter, by what they give us?

Boy   : How should I know? I'm off that religion stuff anyway. Maybe that's why they sent me to see you.

Shrink: Surely you don't think that's the real reason, now do you?

Boy   : I thought doctors were supposed to tell you what was wrong with you and then make you better if they could.

Shrink: (A bit annoyed) Now going round in circles like that isn't going to get us anywhere. Besides, doctors can only help people who want to help themselves. We're not God you know.

Boy : You can say that again. He couldn't even bring me a bloody bike. You couldn't get me a 10 gear bike could you? I could even let you have my 5 gear one 'cause I don't ride it anyway.

Shrink: You've not been to see anyone like me before for help, have you?

Boy : I only know one doctor, Dr Gifford, but my Mum won't take me to see him ever since. . .

Shrink: Yes. . .?

Boy : Since I almost died from my appendix after he said I was trying it on when I wanted help then, but he wouldn't help me.

Shrink: We all make mistakes, even doctors.

Boy : He wouldn't even come to see me at the house and they had to rush me to hospital in a taxi.

Shrink: You mentioned your mother. How do you feel about her?

Boy : The coloured doctor at the hospital said if I had come an hour later I would have had it. He was hopping mad at Dr Gifford.

Shrink: You don't seem to want to talk about your mother. I wonder why not?

Boy : Maybe its because I'd like a new one.

Shrink: (Coughs) Uh, I'm not quite sure what you mean.

Boy : (A bit louder) I said I'd like a new Mum.

Shrink: Perhaps we'd better talk a little more about that?

Boy : I'd like a new Dad too.

Shrink: That's easier said than done. You can't choose new parents like you choose new shoes.

Boy : Who said anything about shoes?

Shrink: You can't even pick your parents first time round. Besides, who would have kept any eye on you when you were too young to look after yourself?

Boy : My Nan would. She's always looked after me anyway.

Shrink: I don't think you want to discuss your mother, or
your father for that matter, but that's all right, we
can move on to something else.

Boy   : They're always fighting and want to get divorced
and they've both got a bit on the side.

Shrink: I think we're beginning to get somewhere now.

Boy   : So why can't I have my 'bit' and get some new
parents then?

Shrink: We're not back to that again, are we?

Boy   : But what about all this stuff about kid's rights? You
can vote now when you're only 18.

Shrink: I'm afraid the law doesn't allow children to pick new
parents like parents go round picking new partners.
Even grown-ups don't have much say on what kind
of kids they have, do they?

Boy   : What if they go and adopt some?

Shrink: That's not the same thing. It's a bit more
complicated than that.

Boy   : Look, if my Mum and Dad decide they want to pair
up with someone else's Dad and Mum, there's
nothing to stop them doing it, right?

Shrink: Uh . . . technically speaking, I suppose not.

Boy   : What do you mean, 'technically'?

Shrink: Well it sort of means that they're legally entitled to
do it, but that doesn't make it right, even though it's
not against the law.

Boy   : So they can go off and get new husbands and new
wives and even new kids, and I can't even get one
lousy new parent, because if I do, I might be
breaking the law.

Shrink: I'm afraid that's the way things are. I don't make the
rules you know and I have to live in the same world
that you do. You'll realize this as you grow older.

Boy   : I wouldn't mind a new brother two. Mine always
knocks me about just 'cause he's bigger than me.

Shrink: You seem to have problems in getting along with lots
of people and not just your parents.

Boy   : All my mates hate their brothers, even their little
ones but they don't go knocking them about.

Shrink: What about their sisters. Do they feel any different
towards them?

Boy   : Yeah, if you got more than one sister you can't be in our gang.

Shrink: That sounds like a funny sort of gang to me. You must really dislike members of the opposite sex and I wonder if that's the reason why you don't want to talk about your mother. Now how does that strike you?

Boy   : You trying to make out I'm a poof or something?

Shrink: (A little taken aback) Uh – no, I simply wondered why you seem to dislike females so much and your mother, after all, is a female; otherwise she wouldn't be your mother, or anyone else's for that matter.

Boy   : If I hated ladies like you're trying to make out, then why would I keep asking if I could have a new mother? I suppose if I kept asking for a new father instead, then you'd be calling me a poof.

Shrink: Uh – I must admit, you seem to have a point there, but getting back to your mother again, it's sometimes the case that boys – or even that men – are too attached to their mothers and this prevents them from forming normal, healthy relationships with other women.

Boy   : You mean like wanting to grab them and get them into bed? That's what we talk a lot about in my gang.

Shrink: Well, at least you appear to be normal in one respect – perhaps a little too normal for your age and I won't quibble about that.

Boy   : So what if I met a nice normal lady who wanted to look after me and I thought she'd make a great Mum when my own Mum didn't want me around anyway? And I wouldn't be bothered about not having a new Dad. I wouldn't even mind if my new Mum was a bit queer as long as she treated me all right.

Shrink: You seem to be more concerned over having a nice mother than a father. I wonder why?

Boy   : Did you have a Mum and Dad around when you were my age?

Shrink: Aren't you avoiding my question?

Boy   : What question?

Shrink: The one about your mother and father.

Boy   : I'm not bothered about either of them; I'd just like a change from the ones I've got. Anyhow, what's wrong with being adopted? I bet you wanted to be adopted before you grew up.

Shrink: As a matter of fact I had a very happy childhood but I hope you'll accept that we're not here to discuss my problems.

Boy   : If you had such a good time when you were a kid why do you have problems now?

Shrink: Everyone has problems. The important thing is to try and solve them. That's why you're here today (slightly stern).

Boy   : Then why won't you let me solve mine? All I want is to be brought up by someone I like and you say there's no way I can have that, just because I'm a kid. Sounds stupid to me.

Shrink: Sometimes it's better to try and cope with a situation than take the easy way out and run away from it. Besides, if you could have a different mother or father, do you think that would be fair to their children if they had any before they met you.

Boy   : My best pal's mother ran off with her boss and nobody asked him or his sister if they thought it was fair to them. At first they had to go and live with some relatives they hated. It was bloody awful and my pal kept running away.

Shrink: Do you think it would really help your friend if he had a new mother?

Boy   : Sure, that's just what happened because last month he got this new step-mum who he thinks is great. His real mother never comes to see him and he doesn't even miss her.

Shrink: A month is not a very long time to see if things will work out or not. It takes a long time before you get to know someone, deep down I mean.

Boy   : Well I've had my own Mum and Dad for 13 years now. That's long enough to find out whether you like someone or whether they like you. If I had kids of my own I wouldn't make them stay with me if they didn't want to. It's not bloody fair.

Shrink: I think you might feel more strongly about your mother and father than you're willing to admit, either to me or to yourself.

Boy : Then why would I keep asking if I could have new parents?

Shrink: Suppose you answer that one yourself?

Boy : Look, if I knew someone my age who didn't like his old man, but I thought his old man was OK and he liked my father better than I did, why couldn't we just do a change round like grown-ups do with each other when they go to parties? You should see what happens at our house on Friday nights after the pubs close!

Shrink: Uh. . . (slightly taken aback) you mean like . . . wife swapping as some people prefer to call it?

Boy : Yeah.

Shrink: Sometimes adults don't behave in sensible ways either.

Boy : Does that mean they have to come and see a doctor like you, just as I have to?

Shrink: Not necessarily.

Boy : Why not?

Shrink: Well, it doesn't follow that you're. . .uh. . .mentally unstable if you're not faithful to your husband or your wife.

Boy : You mean like having a bit of skirt when you should be having if off with your old woman instead?

Shrink: (A bit awkward) I wouldn't put it exactly like that but you're more or less on the right track.

Boy : So grown-ups can go off and leave their kids when they feel like it, but if the kids think their parents are rubbish and want new ones, everyone thinks they're crackers like me.

Shrink: You're pretty good at working out the logic but life isn't as straightforward as you make it to be. What you're suggesting sounds a little 'off beat' to me. Don't you agree?

Boy : Do you think I'm crackers? That social worker they sent round said I was.

Shrink: We don't use words like that here.

Boy   : Well she did and I told her to push off. That's
        probably why I'm here. But if I'm not 'crackers' like
        she said I was, what would you call me then?
Shrink: Someone who doesn't want to discuss his feelings
        towards his mother.
Boy   : Jeez, I've already told you what's bugging me, but
        you keep telling me that's the way the cookie
        crumbles and there's nothing you can do about it.
        Some doctor you are. I'd be better off with Dr
        Gifford.
Shrink: If it helps you to get angry with me, that's all right,
        as long as you realize why you're feeling that way.
Boy   : Who said anything about getting angry?
Shrink: There's nothing wrong with ventilating your
        feelings. Most people are afraid to let themselves go.
Boy   : Are you?
Shrink: Am I what?
Boy   : Afraid to tell anyone just where to shove it when you
        feel like it.
Shrink: There's a time and place for everything.
Boy   : Then it's about time they changed the bloody law
        then and let me have some new parents. That's what
        I said to that social worker when she called me
        'crackers'. She really got mad when I asked her if
        she was wearing a bra. My Nan said she was one of
        those women libbers who don't want to be mothers
        anyway.
Shrink: Well, even if the law was changed and you could
        choose a new mother as you like to call it, don't you
        think you're too young to be able to handle some-
        thing as big as that?
Boy   : Not on your Nellie!
Shrink: I still don't know how you feel about your own
        mother.
Boy   : Did you like your mother?
Shrink: It won't help solve your problems by trying to avoid
        talking about them, will it?
Boy   : I thought you were here to cure me of whatever's
        wrong with me.
Shrink: (Annoyed) I can't do that if you won't tell me what's
        bothering you, now can I?

Boy : But I've told you what's bothering me and you've said that you can't do much about it. It's all right for you, you had a nice Mum and Dad when you were my age. I bet you had a good bike too!

Shrink: (Defensive) What I said was that I had a happy childhood. I didn't say I had a nice mother or father. As a matter of fact I never even knew my father. My mother raised me on her own. And the bike I had didn't even have gears!

Boy : My Mum once told me that my Dad wasn't my real Dad, which is why he never liked me much. So I guess you could say I never knew my Dad either.

Shrink: I think you may be starting to open up now. That's very good. Go on please.

Boy : But if my 'Dad' isn't my real Dad, then no one would mind if I looked for another bloke to take his place.

Shrink: Now you're trying to avoid talking about your problem again, which I'm afraid won't get us much further. Just because your words seem to make sense doesn't necessarily mean that you've chosen the wisest course of action.

Boy : I don't see why I should worry about my Dad if he isn't my real Dad to begin with. You're lucky, you didn't have any 'father' to worry about, but I bet your mother had a few blokes you didn't know about.

Shrink: Lots of boys like you wish they had fathers, even if they weren't their real ones. It's who brings you up that counts and not who brought you into the world!

Boy : Did you wish you had a father. I mean one that you knew, even though he messed around with other women and never had time to play with you?

Shrink: (Slightly exasperated) I'd like to get back to talking about you if you don't mind. Discussing any problems I might have had when I was your age isn't necessarily going to help you. Besides, it was a long time ago — I've almost forgotten how long.

Boy : You don't look that old. How old are you anyway?

Shrink: I'm not as young as you think; in fact I'm probably even old enough to be your father.

Boy   : It would be funny if you really were, since my Mum
         says another man she used to know is my real Dad.
         You never went out with my Mum, did you? She
         was a smasher when she first got married. And I
         once found those nude pictures my old man took of
         her before they got hitched. You sure you never met
         my Mum?

Shrink: Uh – I don't believe so. What makes you say that
         anyway?

Boy   : Well, before I came along, she had a job cleaning the
         doctors' rooms at the big hospital in town, and I
         once heard her telling the lady next door what randy
         buggars the young housemen were, but knowing
         my Mum, it might have been the other way round.
         You never worked at that hospital before you came
         here, did you?

Shrink: Uh, pardon?

Boy   : (Louder) I said did you work there before you started
         pill-pushing here?

Shrink: (Uncomfortably) I think I did spend about three
         months there, filling in for another doctor who was
         off sick, but it was only part-time and the occasional
         week-end.

Boy   : That's when my Mum worked there, on week-ends
         I mean. When I come next time I'll bring a picture of
         her when she was young. She's not so bad-looking
         even now. You'd probably recognize her, although
         she keeps changing her hair colour.

Shrink: I don't think it's necessary to bring any photos of
         your mother. She might not appreciate it (said a bit
         sternly).

Boy   : Maybe you'd like to see a picture of my old man too,
         although he's gone all bald now. I hope I don't go
         bald like him, but maybe I won't if my real Dad had
         lots of hair like you.

Shrink: Perhaps we should get back to talking about you
         again? Otherwise we'll be wasting our time.

Boy   : I thought that's what we've been doing up to now.
         You keep asking about my parents and when I try
         and tell you about them you blame me for not saying
         the right things. I wish you'd make up your mind.

Shrink: (Definitely annoyed) I don't think I put it quite like that. What I'm trying to do is to find out what's bothering you and then give you the opportunity to let me know how you feel about it. Now that's not too difficult to understand, is it? I get the feeling that for an intelligent boy you're being deliberately thick.

Boy : That's just what my Mum says before she belts me.

Shrink: I beg your pardon?

Boy : You're not going to belt me, are you?

Shrink: (Very therapeutic) Is that what you expect from adults? Not everyone is hostile you know.

Boy : You look mad enough to belt me.

Shrink: I'm not angry or 'mad' as you put it, but you may be reacting to me like you react to other grown ups close to you. Did you ever think of it that way?

Boy : I still think you'd like to belt me. I bet you don't like me.

Shrink: (Suppressing anger) Perhaps we could agree that I don't like what you're doing – that is, trying to make me angry with you. But not liking what you're doing isn't the same as not liking you as a person. Can you appreciate the difference?

Boy : You mean you go around liking people when you feel like belting them one. I thought I'm the one who's supposed to be 'crackers'.

Shrink: (Resigned) Perhaps we could move on to something else if you don't mind?

Boy : I don't mind, but when I tell you what I'm thinking about, you make me talk about something else, and when I don't say what you want me to say, you complain that I'm trying to change the subject. I don't know what to say now.

Shrink: How about the first thing that comes into your mind?

Boy : Are you going to show me any of those pictures with those funny inkblots on them and make me tell you what they remind me of? I saw a film like that once where they showed these pictures to a bloke that raped his best friend's wife.

Shrink: Uh. . . . I'm afraid we don't use those sort of techniques here. Perhaps you could tell me something else that comes to mind now?

Boy   : Could I ask you another question?

Shrink: If you must.

Boy   : Do you have any kids?

Shrink: Asking me personal questions like that isn't going to get us anywhere either, but if you must know I have three by my. . .uh. . .first marriage.

Boy   : No kidding?

Shrink: (Slightly cocky) So I probably know a bit more about children than you think I do. I wasn't born yesterday you know.

Boy   : Do you like your kids or do you wish they were never born sometimes?

Shrink: Nobody likes their children all of the time but that doesn't mean they don't love them. You might think about that when you're talking about wanting a new mother or father. Perhaps they're not able to show how much they care for you?

Boy   : I wish my old man was a doctor. Then I could go to a posh school and have a new bike.

Shrink: It doesn't follow that just because someone has a doctor for a father, or even a teacher or accountant for that matter, that it automatically makes him a good parent to his children.

Boy   : I bet you'd make a great father! At least you sit down and talk to kids and listen to what they have to say, even though you keep telling them to say something else.

Shrink: But that's what I've been trained to do. It takes a long time and you've got to do a lot of studying. You've even got to go to university as well. But having a university education is no guarantee that one is going to be a good parent. Many people who've been to university turn out to be rotten parents. I know, because we see lots of their kids here, but we won't go into that now. You're very clever at changing the subject for someone so young.

Boy   : Do you think I could go to university and do a job like yours?

Shrink: I don't see why not, provided you work hard, although I see from your school report (looks down at papers) that you're a bit of a trouble-maker and don't try very hard. You'll never get into a university that way. You'll be lucky if they let you wash up in the university canteen the way you've been carrying on.

Boy : My Mum used to work in a university canteen. She said that the professors were just as randy as the doctors, but she must have liked it there because she stayed for three years before our Sarah came along.

Shrink: (Slightly exasperated) I think we've spent enough time talking about your mother's career or, should I say, avoiding talking about what's really bothering you deep down.

Boy : You wouldn't like to be my Dad would you?

Shrink: Eh???

Boy : Or if you couldn't take on the job, maybe you know some other doctors like you who don't have any kids but would like some.

Shrink: You can't be serious? Besides, that really wouldn't solve any of your problems which you don't seem very willing to talk about anyway.

Boy : Maybe, next time, I could ask my Mum to come along and she could tell you all about me when I was a baby because I can't remember much before I was six or seven. My Nan says I even forget what I've got up to the day before, especially when I've been bad, like when I hid under her bed when she was having it off with the gas-man.

Shrink: (Looks distinctly uncomfortable) Uh – I've had a thought. As we don't appear to be getting very far, perhaps we should give things a rest for a while and I'll send for you if I feel there's anything further that I can do. Sometimes, in fact quite often, it happens that people sort themselves out far better when left to their own devices than when they come along for long chats with someone like myself. Now how does that sound to you?

Boy : Fine by me but I wanted you to meet my Mum. You'd probably like her. Most blokes do.

Shrink: Never mind, I might one day, it's a small world you
        know and it's often funny how things turn out. Very
        funny indeed.
Boy   : Anyway, look after yourself. . .Frank – you said I
        could call you Frank.
Shrink: That's right Andy, take care now and you'll do all
        right. And don't forget to pull your socks up at
        school.
Boy   : I'll try Frank, but by the way. . .
Shrink: What now Andy, I've got another patient waiting.
Boy   : I'm glad they call you Frank.
Shrink: Why's that?
Boy   : My old man's called Frank and I'll think of you every
        time I speak to him although we don't talk much
        these days.
Shrink: (With emotion) Thanks Andy, so long for now.
Boy   : Yeah, so long Frank, see you around sometime.

(Sound of door closing)

ARTHUR KAUFMANN
Sheffield

Mary Jane

What is the matter with Mary Jane?
She's crying with all her might and main
And she won't eat her dinner – rice pudding again –
What *is* the matter with Mary Jane?

What is the matter with Mary Jane?
I've promised her dolls and a daisy chain,
And a book about animals – all in vain
What *is* the matter with Mary Jane?

What is the matter with Mary Jane?
She's perfectly well, and she hasn't a pain;
But, look at her, now she's beginning again –
What *is* the matter with Mary Jane?

What is the matter with Mary Jane?
I've promised her sweets and a ride in the train
And I've begged her to stop for a bit and explain –
What *is* the matter with Mary Jane?

What is the matter with Mary Jane?
She's perfectly well and she hasn't a pain,
And it's lovely rice pudding for dinner again!,
What *is* the matter with Mary Jane?

A. A. Milne: When We Were Very Young

So what are you trying to tell us? That she doesn't like rice pudding, huh! But she doesn't say that for fear of the consequences, because it's not on to not like rice pudding? And I suppose, anyway, the crying gets her out of the rice pudding. Seems reasonable. Hey, I've got loads of patients like that. They don't really say what's the matter, they just complain of this and that; sore backs, sore tummies, headaches. You're lucky, you saw the association with that rice pudding. It takes me ages to sort out what it is that my patients don't like, that makes them whinge.

Course, I know what to do, though. If I'd had Mary Jane seeing me about this crying I'd have explored with her the circumstances that make her feel down, found out about the rice pudding, exploded myths about rice pudding (lumpy, slimy etc) and explained how she could be honest with her parents about what it is she really wants for pudding! Two or three hour-long sessions and I could have put Mary Jane right. Hmmm. Seems a lot of work, and she's already getting what she wants. Better check the textbooks and see that I've got this right.

Now, what would we call Mary Jane? Let's see. Somatizers? No not really; she's certainly manipulative, I expect we could call her DSM-III borderline personality disorder. That's certainly a great help to us. Still, doesn't quite seem my kind of approach. What did old Sigmund say about this. . . Oh yes it's all down to your parents messing up your life and making you feel you can't masturbate. Fair enough, but he'd have taken years to sort out what Milne got

in twenty lines. There's got to be a simpler way. What books
have I got here, now? *Domestic Medicine, or A Treatise on the
Prevention and Cure of Diseases by Regimen and Simple Medicines.*
I haven't seen this for ages. Author, William Buchan M.D.
(M.D. eh? He must know a thing or two) Published 1797 15th
edition. 15th! This has got to be good. Well it's older than
most of my books, but then my Bailey and Love is almost as
old and I don't think surgery has changed that much.

M for manipulation. . . nothing there. N for nervous
diseases. . . H for hysteria and Hypochondriac affections!
*'This difeafe generally attacks the indolent, the luxurious, the
unfortunate and the ftudious. If becomes daily more common in this
country, owing, no doubt, to the increafe of luxury and fedentary
employments'.* Wonderful! That's just the sort of person A. A.
Milne always wrote about. So this man Buchan has got the
demography right, what about the treatment?

*'Hypochondriac perfons ought never to faft long, and their food
should be folid and nourifhing'.* Hmm. Could be difficult with
Mary Jane, what with her food fads, but it might help some
of my lot. *'All acefcent and windy vegetables are to be avoided.
Flefh meats agree best with them, and their drink fhould be old claret
or good madeira. Should thefe difagree with the ftomach, water with
a little brandy or rum in it may be drank.'* Gosh, I wish I'd known
about this when I worked in Oxford; not so useful in Moss
Side! Here we go, though. . . *'Exercife of every kind is ufeful.
The cold bath is likewife beneficial and, where it does not agree with
the patient, frictions with the flefh-brufh or a coarfe cloth may be
tried.'* Well, I think he's got something for me here. Cold
baths is about all most of mine can afford! *'If the patient has
it in his power, he ought to travel either by fea or land. A voyage
or a long journey, efpecially towards a warmer climate, will be of
more fervice than any medicine.'* How else would the denizens
of 18th century England have travelled, I wonder?

I'm just wondering what physiological basis he's using for
these treatments. *'The general intentions of cure, in this difease,
are to ftrengthen the alimentary canal, and to promote the
fecretions'.* . . . Sorry? . . . *'different preparations of iron and
peruvian bark. . . after proper evacuations. If the patient be coftive,
it will be neceffary to make ufe of fome gentle opening medicine, as
pills compofed of equal parts of aloes, rhubarb and afafoetida. . .
such as cannot bear the afafoetida may fubftitute Spanish foap in its*

place.' Well, that seems straightforward. But I was still wondering if we could have got it so wrong; you see, we thought that these simple remedies didn't get to the heart of the matter. . . *'nervous affections arife more frequently from caufes, which it is in a great meafure in our own power to avoid, than from difeafes or an original fault in the conftitution. Exceffive grief, intenfe ftudy, improper diet, and the neglect or exercife are the great sources of this extenfive clafs of difeafes.'*

Well, that's all right then. As I underftand it, (sorry, understand it), he's saying that we could avoid being somatizers but if we do get it then a good dose of the salts should put it right. Hooray for William. But what would you say was the biggest contributing factor to hypochondriac affections?. . .

' . . .indolence. The active and laborious are feldom troubled with them. They are referved for the children of eafe and affluence, who generally feel their keeneft force. All we fhall fay to fuch perfons is that the means of prevention and cure are both in their own power. If the conftitution of man is fuch that he muft either labour or fuffer difeafes, surely no individual has any right to expect an exemption from the general rule.'

So it's a case of pull yourself together, by the look of it. Snap out of it, get yourself back to work and stop whining. You wouldn't have got a sick note out of W. Buchan M.D., so you're not getting one out of me. I must say this approach appeals to me. I wonder if he's got any more good advice for an inner city GP. We see a lot of alcoholism, a lot of depression around here.

Of Melancholy

'Melancholy is that fate of alienation or weaknefs of the mind which renders people incapable of enjoying the pleafures, or performing the duties of life. It is a degree of infanity, and often terminates in abfolute madnefs.'

Causes

'It may proceed from an hereditary difpofition; intenfe thinking, efpecially where the mind is long occupied about one object; violent paffions or affections of the mind, as love, fear, joy, grief, pride and

fuch like. It may alfo be occafioned by exceffive venery; narcotic or ftupefactive poifons; a fedentary life; folitude; the suppreffion of cuftomary evacuations; acute fevers, or other difeafes. To all of which we may add gloomy or miftaken notions of religion.' Well we may, William, but what about the treatment? Oh all right then, the symptoms.

'The body is generally bound; the urine thin and in small quantity, the ftomach and the bowels inflated with wind; the complexion pale; the pulse slow and weak. The functions of the mind are alfo greatly perverted in fo much that the patient often imagines himfelf dead, or changed into fome other animal. Some have imagined their bodies were made of glafs, or other brittle fubftances and were afraid to move, left they fhould be broken to pieces. The unhappy patient in this cafe, unlefs carefully watched, is apt to put an end to his own miferable life.'

Yes, but the treatment, Bill, the treatment!

'The diet fhould confift chiefly of vegetables of a cooling and opening quality. Animal food, efpecially falted or fmoke-dried fifh or flefh fhould be avoided. All kinds of fhellfifh are bad. . . Boerhaave gives an inftance of a patient who, by a long use of whey, water, and garden fruit, recovered, after having evacuated a great quantity of black coloured matter.'

I think I'm getting the hang of it now. There's not a great deal between Dr Buchan and holistic practitioners of the present day. 'You are what you eat' seems to be the cry. If you insist on feasting on salt-dried fish, it's not surprising you end up feeling like one, and loafing about the place feeling depressed and concealing in your lumina a great deal of black coloured matter. I'm going to lend this book to our dietitian. Her role would be instantly enhanced. Diet sheets would be revolutionized. I, in my turn, will cry in alarm to the next patient with a GHQ score of 15 through the door, 'you've been at the fish again!' But I interrupt you, sir.

Medicine

'When the patient is in a low ftate, his mind ought to be foothed and diverted with variety of amufements, as entertaining ftories, paftimes, mufic, etc. This feems to have been the method of curing melancholy among the Jews, as we learn from the ftory of King Saul; and indeed it is a very rational one. When the patient is high,

evacuations are neceffary. In this cafe he muft be bled, and have his body kept open by purging medicines, as manna, rhubarb, cream of tartar, or the soluble tartar. I have feen the laft have very happy effects.' Very happy for who, one wonders? Given the propensity of the profession at this time for opening medicines, and given the state of public sanitation at the time of the industrial revolution, I would not be at all surprised if a number of the rest of the household became quite melancholic after a week or two of this lot. But you were saying. . .?

'Were he forced to ride or walk a certain number of miles every day, it would tend greatly to alleviate his disorder; but it would have ftill a better effect, if he were obliged to labour a piece of ground. By digging, hoeing, planting, sowing &c. both the body and the mind would be exercifed. A plan of this kind, with a ftrict attention to diet is a much more rational method of cure than confining the patient indoors and plying him with medicines.' Quite; he could plant some rhubarb for a start. Now I come to think about, Dr Buchan is only using a little ploy I've used for years; I'm always wittering on about the mind-body link. So much so that I've quite forgotten that it works both ways. *Mens sana in corpore sano.* He's saying that if your mind is bit out of order it's because your body is all down the shute. And he goes further. If the bottom's fallen out of your world, make the world fall out of your bottom!

I like this man. He says what he thinks and to hell with the evidence. No controlled trials for him, no anxieties about matching for social class, age and sex. On the other hand, listen to this: *'Whenever I had in it in my power to place them under the care of proper nurfes, to infruct these nurfes in their duty, and to be fatisfied that they performed it, very few of them died; but when, from diftance of place, and other unavoidable circumftances, the children were left to the fole care of mercenary nurfes, without any perfon to infruct or fuperintend them, fcarce any of them lived.'* And you don't get evidence like that these days. As for references, *'I have not troubled the reader with a ufelefs parade of quotations from different authors, but have in general adopted their obfervations where my own were defective, or totally wanting.'* You try using that on the BMJ referees. Here is a man after (actually before) the heart of Sir Lancelot Spratt, of Bargepole.

Incidentally, they both like a tipple; how is that with you,
Dr Buchan?

'*Temperance may juftly be called the parent of health; yet numbers
of mankind act as if they thought difeafes and death too flow in their
progress, and by intemperance and debauch feem, as it were, to
folicit their approach.*' Intemperance and debauch, eh? What
about a dram now and again then. '*Every act of intoxication
puts nature to the expense of a fever, in order to difcharge the
poifonous draught. When this is repeated almoft every day, it is eafy
to forefee the confequences.*' But a nip now and again, surely that
would . . .? '*Many people injure their health by drinking, who
feldom get drunk. The continual habit of foaking, as it is called,
though its effects be not fo violent, is not lefs pernicious. When the
veffels are kept conftantly full and upon the ftretch, the different
digeftions cannot be properly performed, nor the humours prepared.
Hence moft people of this character are afflicted with the gout, the
gravel, ulcerous sores on the legs, &c.*' Crikey. It's these &cs
which get to me. Got any advice for us, Doctor? What, none?
There's not a word about the treatment of alcoholism in the
whole book! And I thought you knew the lot. But here's a
gem; a hair-of-the-dog like none you've ever had.

'*A young man, about fifteen years of age, had, for a hire, drank
ten glaffes of ftrong brandy. He soon fell faft afleep and continued
in that fituation for feveral hours, till at length his uneafy manner
of breathing, the coldnefs of his extremities and other threatening
symptoms, alarmed his friends and made them fend for me. . ..I
tried to roufe him, but in vain, by pinching, shaking, applying
volatile fpirits to his nose. A few ounces of blood were taken from his
arm, and a mixture of vinegar and water was poured into his mouth;
but as he could not fwallow very little of this got into his ftomach.
I ordered his leg to be put into warm water and a sharp clyfter to
be immediately adminiftered. This gave him a ftool and was the firft
thing that relieved him. It was afterwards repeated with the same
happy effect, and feemed to be the chief caufe of his recovery.*' If
Dr Buchan went home without having gazed upon a number
of stools he would have not slept well in his bed. He was a
stool-gazer of the first degree.

Well, what have we learnt? I'll tell you what I've learnt;
stop pussy-footing around with mental illness and dole out
the advice and the medicine. Psychotherapy, forget it.
Counselling, goodbye. Welcome my good friends dogmatic

advice and asafoetida. Fifteen editions say they're not wrong.

'Hello, do come in and sit down. . ..How has Mary Jane been since I saw you last?. . . . Oh, that is disappointing. . . . Well, I've been talking to some colleagues who know a bit about these things and I've read up a bit about Mary Jane's problems. I was just wondering. . . . how are her bowels?'

ANDREW PROCTER
Gainsborough

7 Psychology

You have to know how to deal with foreigners in my neck of the woods because we have a lot of them going through the lab. This Venezuelan visiting scientist came up to me one day and said 'You are clinician. I have pain in side.' 'Left side or right side?' I asked. 'Back side,' he replied.

And once, we had a visit from the Armenian Minister of Health, clutching the tattered remains of the English he picked up long ago as a young postgraduate student in Glasgow. As we toasted each other at our farewell dinner, he tried – and failed – to recall the expression, 'Bottoms up,' and burst forth delightedly with 'I toast you up your bottom!'

But Americans are always with us and the most memorable by far, the brashest by far, was Carl Philip Emanuel Fink. Not Wilhelm Friedmann, not Johann Christoph but CPE, and it is ironic that he was tone deaf. He displayed one of those American Masonic rings as big as a pigeon's egg and used to go around telling everybody that his IQ was 180. 'Is that fahrenheit or centigrade?', my sharp, little secretary asked him innocently. His special interest was psychiatric genetics and he spent much time making chromosome preparations from cell cultures of his own mouth scrapings. One morning, he emerged from the lab, pale and worried and said, 'I think I'm tetraploid.' Just for a moment it seemed possible – this homunculus, crazed with a superabundance of Jewish genes – but the answer was technical and he returned to the States, to live happily ever after at the National Institute of Mental Health.

Counselling in Terminal Care

Bill was a corporation dust cart driver, Edith his dutiful, typically Lancastrian wife. They lived in a tiny terraced house nestling close to the vulgar sprawl of the airport. They loved their little house. Even the hustle and bustle of the adjacent airport made very little intrusion into their close-knit family life.

Bill smoked heavily – Capstan's – and how Edith hated their smell, preferring the diesel fumes spewing out of the BA111s flying in onto the runway, often it seemed only a few yards overhead. They seemed to live like this, each holding extreme views and adopting habits at variance with the other. They agreed to my mind, only on one thing, the fortunes of Manchester City FC (we never mentioned United).

My main concern was always for Bill's lungs – he had chronic bronchitis – a legacy from the 'dreaded weed'. Latterly I came to visit regularly as he became increasingly housebound. Edith, always the picture of health, always positive in her attitude to life, suddenly took ill. Eventually it became obvious she was very ill. Carcinoma of the uterus. With secondaries.

I well remember on that hot June day when she was discharged from the Christie Hospital, leaning against the gable end outside wall of their little house chatting to their daughter, Janet. I warned her of the specialists' predictions that her mother could have no more than three months to live. 'Do you think,' I asked 'that you could break the news gently to your father?' 'Then he might in time tell your mother.' We agreed.

Six months later, after going into a complete remission (on drugs) Edith was up and about, shopping and cooking as usual. So much for the gloomy prediction!

It had become obvious from the start that Edith fully appreciated the diagnosis and the probable poor outcome, but had brushed aside the whole episode, in her usual phlegmatic way. It was never mentioned again.

Later I had occasion to meet her daughter. 'How in fact did our attempts at terminal counselling work?' I asked. 'Well,' said Janet, 'I did tell Dad'. When he broached the subject with Edith she agreed she was quite aware of the seriousness of her illness. 'Yes, of course I know,' she said. 'Well,' Bill had replied, 'don't you think we should prepare – er – prepare for it?' 'For what, damn you?' Edith retorted. Long pause. 'Well,' said Bill, gathering strength and momentum, 'where would you like to be buried?' 'On top of you,' replied Edith, as quick as a flash. End of conversation.

And she will be. Bill died last year.

EGRYN M. JONES
Wilmslow

Psychological Aspects of Flatulence: The Heart of the Matter

We ate hard, we drank much;
We expelled our airs where we stood.
We were happy; our hearts were free,
Never to be confined again.

Excretius, c. 150 BC

Introduction

Despite modern advances in the diagnosis and treatment of cardiovascular disease, it is remarkable there has been such little recognition of the importance of psychological aspects of flatulence in our understanding of heart disorders. In this article we shall attempt to explore some of the relationships between flatulence and personality and how such factors affect the workings of this vital organ. We shall also explore the role of the family doctor as well as prospects for research in this largely neglected area of human activity.

In doing so, we make no claim of adding to the totality of human knowledge, for we are simply rediscovering 'scientifically' what has been subjectively experienced by Man (as well as many simpler forms of life) since the evolution of the very first functional anus. For example, the sudden release of wind otherwise referred to as 'gas' by our American colleagues will often result in a lowering of blood pressure, with no adverse side effects unless, of course, the diastolic pressure is abnormally depressed to begin with (Airman, 1972). Thus, encouraging patients who are at risk of coronary artery disease to let off 'healthful vapours' – at least once every hour – is likely to be beneficial in the long run, not to mention the lowering of anxiety gained in the process.

Even when in company or in a delicate social situation such as the near completion of a conquest of a member of the opposite gender when the inhibition of rectal vapours in combination with sexual excitement may cause a dangerous rise in blood pressure (Lecher, 1985), there may be considerable danger to life itself if there is no opportunity to relieve one's self accordingly – particularly in cases where there is a long-standing family history of heart disease. The association between cardiovascular problems and temperament has long since been recognized. However, what has been lacking until recently are correlational studies of noise levels arising from the act of flatulence itself and the personality of the individual flatulator.

Current Investigations and Exploratory Studies

Recent pilot studies (Bottomly, 1987) have suggested that those of an introverted nature are, on average, more likely to expel relatively quiet emissions when say, compared with those of a more outgoing or extroverted disposition, who may actually enjoy 'letting off' in public as a means of either gaining attention or even embarrassing those around them. In about four percent of those who fall into the 'letting off' catagory, the frequency of emissions may reach the level of an actual perversion, thereby leading to a number of adverse social consequences, including grievous bodily harm to the emitters themselves.

Should such anti-social extrovert behaviour persist, it will be necessary to refer the patient to a psychiatrist with a particular interest in this area, preferably one specializing in the Freudian treatment of those unfortunates who, during the course of infant development, have fixated at the anal stage. On the other hand, the introvert's persistent attempts to minimize what he perceives as unacceptable flatulence will almost certainly exacerbate tendencies to angina, tachycardia or even imaginary thoughts that all is not well with cardiovascular function. In such instances it may be advisable for the sufferer to join a psychotherapy group where more 'assertive' or extrovert-emission behaviour may be actively encouraged albeit not beyond anti-social limits; otherwise as has already been pointed out psychiatric complications may arise.

With growing public awareness of the importance of roughage in proper bowel function, it is not surprising to learn that advocates of the 'Flatulence Always Releases Tension' movement have formed themselves into voluntary cardiogaseous groups, known nationally in their abbreviated form as FART. Lately there has been talk of even forming a specialist subsidiary section for doctors interested in cardio-proctological problems, under the guise of MEDIFART. If all goes according to plan it is envisaged that FART and MEDIFART (F and MF) will soon combine forces to sponsor research into the complex interactions between flatulence and cardiovascular function, which has been long overdue, not to mention much needed studies between factors such as chest-spasm and constipation in the over 40s (Dungworth, 1988).

Already, there are proposals afoot to set up fellowships for study amongst the inhabitants of the Wrectal cult of Southeast Siberia who regard both frequency and volume of anal aerations as an important sign of social status – as well as a necessary prophylactic measure against stroke in all its forms. Moreover, it is of some concern to the present government that the Russians are leaps and bounds ahead in this vital area of scientific enquiry.

The Role of the Family Doctor

Family doctors are in an unique position to educate their patients towards 'positive' flatulence, including the mechanism of belching as well as the more socially sensitive anal exhalations. When, for example, listening to the patient's chest, it can be helpful for the physician to let off wind at the same time, thereby teaching the patient to associate the doctor's soothing hands and voice with the act of flatulence itself. This technique is especially useful with patients of a very inhibited nature, who can gradually be 'desensitized' to what they fear as the potentially punitive attitudes of society towards breaking wind in public – or even in private – amongst consenting adults who have forsaken free love in favour of virtually infection-free, free flatulence.

It may also be helpful for the doctor to try and belch when breaking wind, albeit preferably when there has been no ingestion of large quantities of curry or garlic the night before. In addition, notices and pamphlets extolling both the benefits and the pleasures of passing intestinal and stomach gases should be prominently displayed in the surgery waiting room, even by way of photos of pretty models in suspenders and black stockings, posing in obvious states of animated pleasure as they demonstrate their intestinal motions of relief and delight (La Rue, 1984).

Case Study 1

Miss Ida X, a 59 year-old virgin spinster, consulted her doctor on the fourth Tuesday of each month because of chest pains. Repeated clinical examination plus hospital investigation failed to reveal any organic cause for her complaint and psychological causation was strongly suspected. But after 13 years of surgery attendances, her long-patient doctor, who was listening to her chest, suddenly broke wind, which caused Miss X to faint on the spot in extreme embarrassment. As she fell the doctor's stethoscope caught up in her bra strap causing the said garment to become totally detached and then propelled out of the open window of the examining room on to a passing lorry, never to be seen again.

During the course of Miss X's faint the doctor failed to notice her loss of attire and, for reasons which remain obscure to this day, decided to give mouth-to-mouth resuscitation. When Miss X finally came round, she assumed that her doctor (whom she had secretly been in love with for the past 13 years) could no longer contain his feelings for her, since he was not only kissing her with heavy breaths but also had her down on the floor, bare-breasted and all.

Unfortunately, the doctor's notes for the particular consultation went missing but, suffice to say, Miss X no longer complained of chest pains on subsequent visits, thereby demonstrating the effect of breaking wind, albeit by proxy, on complaints of pain arising from the region of the heart and adjoining structures. She also decided to burn her remaining bras.

Sadly, the doctor concerned had to leave the practice for medical/psychiatric reasons although Miss X subsequently went on to become an active member of FART, raising considerable amounts of money at jumble sales and fêtes by way of sales of prune jam – which she hoped would help to break down the prohibitions against breaking wind in neighbourhood surgeries, thereby encouraging rapport between patients and doctors.

Case Study 2

Mr Leonard Z, married, aged 49, suffered with nervous flatulence since the age of 19 when he first met his wife. Initially it was thought that this was due to 'nerves' associated with the early stages of romantic attraction. However, when the frequency of wind-breaks increased to about one every 30 seconds (when they were on honeymoon), he finally sought medical help. A number of gastrointestinal preparations were prescribed but none resulted in any noticeable decrease in the frequency of flatulation which, during both waking and sleep, averaged out to 2880 emissions each 24 hour period, or probably well beyond the one per cent level of statistical significance, even in the absence of reliable 'normative' data.

In desperation, Mr Z sought help from a private alternative medicine clinic, specializing in the treatment of chronic colonic disorders by cocoa butter massage. As luck would have it he soon fell in love with his 'therapist', an 18 year-old former beauty queen whose appetite for the physical side of love far exceeded his. Their relationship continued for three months until such time as his efforts to satisfy this therapist's needs resulted in a massive coronary, eventually requiring by-pass surgery. However, to the surprise of everyone including the local proctological society, his flatulence suddenly ceased. Unfortunately he succumbed before further investigation could shed more light on the obviously complex relationships between coronary function and flatulence as well as how such factors are affected by frequency of sexual intercourse in combination with cocoa butter absorption in middle-aged males.

Discussion

Whilst investigations into flatulence and heart disease are still in their early stages, there seems little doubt that passing wind can have an important bearing on cardiac efficiency in association with a number of psychological factors. In this article, we have described how the release of intestinal gases may have a direct effect on lowering blood pressure, which could well prove one of the most significant discoveries in cardiovascular function since that of the circulation of the blood itself. We have also sought to demonstrate the importance of personality type in relation to flatulating behaviour and how this might account for a higher incidence of cardiac disorders in those of a more introverted disposition. Indeed, this factor might even partially account for the susceptibility of the medical profession to premature heart attacks.

Although many studies have been carried out over the years on heart disease in relation to psychological factors, it is only recently that the physical role of flatulence has come to the fore; no doubt, it will soon be regarded as having increasing relevance in a wide range of cardiac as well as other kinds of disorder. The role of the family doctor in educating the public as to the healthful aspects of flatulence cannot be emphasized sufficiently. The neighbourhood practitioner is in the front line in the never-ending battle against heart disease and, in effect, the campaign to make 'anal exhalations' socially and psychologically acceptable.

If doctors have been successful in reducing tobacco smoke emissions amongst their patients, they must be equally vigorous in encouraging them to flatulate instead. There seems little sense in improving cardiac health by stopping someone smoking only to allow him or her to suppress 'natural' emissions because of repressive and outdated social mores affecting the lower end of the alimentary canal. Despite the relative lack of normative studies on the actual frequency of flatulence behaviour – as well as over-reliance on anecdotal reports – the evidence thus far suggests that a great deal more effort and research funding will have to be put into this area of study, especially as it applies to cardiovascular illness. Fortunately, the lay public through its increasing interest and support for FART is totally behind the medical profession in its urgent attempts to elucidate the complex web of factors between heart function, the inner workings of the mind and the nature of flatulence itself.

One exciting area of ongoing research is the fitting of individual flatulence meters to university student volunteers, so as to provide some form of 'base line' as to the frequency, intensity and decibel rating of 'wind-breaks' in this particular age group. Preliminary analyses on some 5000 subjects suggests a small but significant relationship between such factors as gender and field of study (e.g. with female sociology students topping the list) as well as between heart rate and level of self-awareness that a flatulatory act has actually occurred. There is also exciting talk of a combined pacemaker/flatulence recorder which can be linked by a miniature transformer to a central computer, thereby offering instant analysis of data received simultaneously from virtually thousands of individuals. The implications here for advancing the scope of medical and psychological studies almost seem to defy description. Indeed, the heat and gases emitted from the bowel itself might be utilized to furnish a highly reliable source of energy for pacemakers and, at a stroke, do away with the need for replacement of batteries or reliance on other expensive 'unnatural' sources of power (a point which has met with unanimous favour from conservationist groups of all political complexions).

From a social standpoint the fear of breaking wind in public could well become a thing of the past. No longer would children be admonished for performing a perfectly natural act. The reduction in anxiety and stress in the population as a whole would be enormous, accompanied by almost certain beneficial effects in the cardiovascular systems of millions of potential sufferers.

Professional Issues

Plans are in progress to publish a new journal to assist scientific workers with a special interest in psycho-cardio-flatulatory problems. It is hoped that financial assistance will be forthcoming from various government bodies in order to ease the passage of this new publication into the highly competitive market of medical journalism. It is intended that the journal be read by the intelligent lay audience as well as by interested professionals. So as to attract the widest possible audience it has been decided to call this publication 'Windbreak'. It has also been suggested that an International Conference Centre be built for the specific purpose of providing a much needed focal point for the growing interest in flatulence and cardiac illnesses. Although many financial problems remain to be overcome, there appears to be unanimous agreement that the Centre be cited just outside Windygates in Fife.

Clearly, a great deal remains to be done but, given the interest and enthusiasm generated thus far, there will almost certainly be continuing pressure to achieve what in the end will seem no longer than a few heart beats away.

References

Airman, B.O. (1972) Hypertension and flatulence. *New England Journal of Gaseous Studies*, 18, 232–241.

Bottomly, U.P. (1987) Preliminary studies of flatuo-noise levels and personality type. Unpublished M.A. thesis. Open University.

Dungworth, P.U. (1988) Constipation and impotence. *Virility*, 88, 69. Leading article.

La Rue, Mimi (1984) Personal communication – details supplied on request.

Lecher, F.A. (1985) Sexual attraction and flatulence. *Penthouse Classics*, 12, 49–52.

ARTHUR KAUFMANN
Sheffield

Where Angels Fear to Tread

There is a certain type of person, hard to define, but recognizable in so many ways, with the ability to tread in dogs' messes. They do it unwittingly, seemingly unaware of their feet, the ground they stand on, or the fearful effluvia they incur with every step. Their shoes are invariably brogues with treads like well-worn tractor tyres, and wherever they walk their footprints are like an obscene rubber stamp on the fitted carpets of this life. Worse is to come: for when advised of their predicament, they execute a soft-shoe-shuffle much as a swarm of flies might desecrate the icing on a cake. For the life of me; I don't know why they do it. They're always such *nice* people.

JAMES HENRY PITT-PAYNE
Beckenham

8 Neurology

I mentioned that I am a self-made psychiatrist. In fact, I'm only a psychiatrist by contagion – so I thought a few actual out-patient sessions wouldn't do me any harm. Almost the first patient I saw was this old duck. She said, 'it's lonely being a neurone.' At once, I was at my most charming and sympathetic. 'Well, it needn't be. You can talk to the other neurones. If you're GABAergic, you can inhibit them. . .' She looked at me strangely, 'I said it's lonely being on your own.'

Neurology has progressed massively since I was a young houseman and we now have substantial insights into hypothalamic dysfunction. In those days, however, the Pickwickian fat boy, the subject of the professorial ward round, had to be satisfied with the label 'Froelich's syndrome' or 'dystrophia adiposogenitalis'. My chief, the Professor of Paediatrics, was a great showman and attracted a vast entourage. He was also a bit of a bully and always used to pick on one particular student with an uncanny likeness to Queen Victoria*. 'Look at this boy. Look at his belly. What's your diagnosis, Miss Davidson?' Miss Davidson was petrified. She was hypnotized, like a rabbit transfixed by a car's headlights. She was speechless. 'Come now, Miss Davidson. . .' Miss Davidson took a deep breath, 'Could it be a case of imperforate anus?'

Head-case

*M*y patient was a junior subaltern, and had been lecturing his platoon on the subject of gun safety. He'd dealt with the various parts of the gun, then he had said: 'One vital thing! Never assume that a gun is safe. I know for certain that this gun is not loaded, I have carefully inspected it

---

* *Albert to Victoria*: Ach! So!! There you are, my little monarch of the glen. *Victoria to Albert*: We are not a moose.

myself – but it would be very foolish for me to put it to my head and pull the trigger. Thus.'

Bang! Lump of lead in a frontal lobe.

Now, most people think that if you shoot yourself in the head you're dead, but of course that isn't always so. If you know the right spot – or the wrong spot? – and put a slug in there, it's curtains quick, but there are sizeable chunks of grey matter without which you can manage very nicely. My patient had chanced to select one of the less indispensable areas.

But it is healthier to refrain from carrying mineral deposits around in your cranium for long, so when he was sufficiently recovered to be fit for surgery, my boss decided to open up his skull a bit more than he had contrived to arrange already, and took him down to theatre.

The neuro-theatre was at the far end of a very long corridor (co-incidentally, handy for the cemetery) and, after a trying day, I used to find it a pretty taxing walk, so I kept a battered bike in Casualty. The boss had already got to work dismantling the dome; I, as dogsbody, had to hold the sucker to keep the field of operations as clear as possible of blood and CSF. It wasn't altogether easy as we were working in the confined space of the partially-opened skull, and my chief's hands and instruments constantly blocked my view as I moved the sucker around. Not surprisingly, I presently saw something shooting up the tube that wasn't blood and wasn't CSF.

I called my chief's attention to it: 'I say, sir, there's some brain going up the sucker.' And my chief, God rest his soul, chuckled, and said, in his broad Yorkshire accent, something I've never forgotten in all these many years. 'Oh! Ah wouldn't worry, lad. Ah doan't think he ever uses that bit.'

DENIS CASHMAN
Cullercoats

Neurological Diagnosis

Acneiform, greasy and leathered,
He sat down, he belched and he said,
'Woss this 'orrible lump on me neck, doc?'
I replied, 'It's known as your head.'

Thin End

The anorexic girl grew thinner and thinner,
Which wasn't surprising 'cos nothing went in 'er.
When she died, her friends, in dubious taste,
Shook their heads sadly and said 'What a waist.'

RICHARD WYNDHAM
Marlingford

Driving

Once doctors have qualified, they tend to miss out on some of the more mundane experiences of life. Ask one if he has had to travel on a bus since his final exams, and you may get a variety of responses, including 'Oh, occasionally,' or 'Er, no,' or 'What!?'. In Canada, to the 'what?', will be added, 'You must be joking', or words to that effect. There will be enough emphasis on any or all of those words to imply insanity in the questioner.

Most Canadian families have at least one car, usually two, and many have three. Doctors usually fall into the latter group. Symbolic of their professional prosperity, no doubt, and consistent with the remark of an eminent mentor of mine, who ruefully observed that the success of his orthopaedic colleagues could be measured by the length of the nose of the Rolls Royce that they drove!

This wheeled endowment was also a practical convenience in a country where older children expect to drive to school and wives need one to get to the golf course. The third car was often a banger, and 'last one out in the morning gets it', was the rule.

Unusually for me, I was last out, on the occasion that I am about to describe (and there is a 'nervous' component to this story, if you will bear with me), and it was I that got the banger, which managed to get me to my office, but which could not be persuaded to co-operate for the return journey. Much cursing followed, to myself of course, because naturally there was no one at home, and ergo, no other car. The options were plain. Either get a cab, or 'what the hell, let's try the bus.' I did the latter. First question, 'which bus?'

Simple, you may say, but not in the depth of the prairie winter, where no one hangs around on street corners just to be asked such a damn fool question. For a start, the buses aren't marked as in London – 'take a number 11', and for a second, I didn't want to be recognized.

I eventually chanced my arm, and ascended the steps of a likely looking vehicle, only to find to my further embarrassment, that it was a 'pay as you enter with the correct fare' type. The driver was incredulous when I asked him how much. Probably thought I'd been in gaol, or something. At least he didn't recognize me.

I slunk into a seat at the back, and we started to move, thankfully in the right direction, and I started to relax. No one had seen me, and with a bit of luck I would get home unnoticed.

A few minutes later, I noticed that the young woman in front of me was starting to shake, gently at first, then more vigorously, and then alarmingly, and she fell to the floor in a full blown epileptic fit.

'Oh hell, I don't believe this!' I must pretend not to notice. I can't do anything. Someone else will help. Well, they did. Another young woman crawled along the floor, to proffer assistance, which embarrassed me enough to do the same. We met at the 'patient'. 'It's OK,' she said, 'I'm a nurse.' 'I'm a doctor,' I replied, in a very low whisper.

By this time, the 'patient' was blue, and apparently apnoeic; the bus driver had stopped, and summoned help on his radio, and very soon, the wailing of the rescue service vehicle could be heard. The other passengers were crowding in to what they thought was going to be a juicy drama.

Coincidentally with the arrival of not one, but two ambulances, the young girl started to breath, and become pink again and as several burly men rushed on to the bus, she sat up, and demanded to know what was going on.

Very shortly afterwards, she was in full command, and refusing to go to the hospital. 'I want to carry on, and go home,' she said. 'You can't do that,' said the lead ambulance-man. 'You have to go.' 'I won't!' 'Regulations say that you must!' '*** to the regulations!' There was a stand off.

I had to approach the man, and say that she was probably OK to continue her journey. 'Who the hell are you?,' he said. 'I am a doctor,' I replied, in as low a voice as I could manage. He looked very surprised, but give him his due, he didn't ask the obvious question. 'Well, if you sign here, to say that she is all right, that's fine with me.' 'Your full name and address, Doctor!': this is an exceedingly loud voice.

The game was up by then, so I signed, and he left, and the journey continued, with the young woman perfectly normal again.

I eventually got home. 'Guess what happened to me?' 'Serve you right for going on the bus.' Quite so.

I was telling the tale to my colleagues, the next morning, and one said, 'I know who that was. She's one of mine. Never takes her pills properly. Always having fits. Bloody nuisance she is!' Quite so again.

Six months later, when the banger let my wife down, resulting in an uneventful bus journey for her, I had to buy a new car. There's no justice in this world!

JOHN H. TAYLOR
Lichfield

Neuroanatomy: The Anatomy of a Neurologist

Neurologists are different! They are super specialists in a super speciality. Don't call them nerve doctors. They prefer to be known as 'brain doctors'. The transformation to 'brain doctor' begins soon after graduation. A detailed knowledge of the brain centres and all their connections is required. Your own connections determine your acceptance into brain centres such as Queen's Square or Neurology-upon-Tyne. There you learn complex words from texts with simple titles. '*Brain*.' You discover that the angular gyrus is not a helicopter and the hippocampus is not an African waterhole! Finding your way through the nerve tracts is like becoming a London cabbie. 'Turn left at the circle of Willis, past the pons and down to the medulla.' To this knowledge is added the neurologists' own jargon. The more incomprehensible you are, the more successful you become. In addition to the ubiquitous Hb, ESR, ECG, neurologists have their EMG and EEG. I am sure I once heard a request for an EGG.

A neurological sense of dress develops. Their white coats are always clean (not much blood is spilt on the neurology ward). The coat is offset with a brightly coloured hat pin. This pin is used to test sensation. It is not an instrument of voodoo. Just as army officers carry swagger sticks, the neurologists have their own staff of authority. This is the tendon hammer. All doctors know the instrument but only neurologists can wield it with uniform style. One flick of the stick and the reflexes spring to life. Like Moses striking the rock, a diagnosis spouts forth. Once the diagnosis is made, the patient's problems are not over. Many neurological diseases cannot be cured, but the neurologist remains cheerful. The patient must be entertained until Nature takes its course. With no pressure to save the patient, the junior neurologist enjoys a more relaxed existence than his peers in acute medicine or surgery.

On Monday mornings a hospital mess is like a wartime airfield after a mission. Tired faces, haggard by long hours of duty, stare down at dull breakfasts. Empty places at the table show that, for some, the ordeal is not yet over. 'Where's Smithy this morning?' 'Night Sister got him over Casualty. He never had a chance.'

Into this gloomy scene would stride the neurologist. Bright, alert and well groomed. 'No calls at all! Slept like a log. What's for breakfast?'

If the 'brain doctor' arrived looking as brain dead as everyone else, you knew there must have been a good party the night before!

Oscar Wilde once quipped that the English gentleman foxhunting was 'the unspeakable in pursuit of the uneatable.' Would Wilde have deemed the neurologist to be the unspeakable in pursuit of the untreatable?

JOHN STUART DOWDEN
Naracoorte, Australia

Of Sense and Sensibility

Part of the basic stuff of Neurology are the Senses. How many are there? I recalled that there were five and came up with sight, hearing and touch. After a moment, smell and taste surfaced. But was it seven? Having checked my own skull and hands I had to look it up – the seven included speech and articulation as extras. With these, however, the circle widened disconcertingly. What about the notorious sense of shame, that elusive sense of humour and good old reliable common sense? (I'm not at all sure anyone knows what common sense is, although, like a sense of humour, we would all claim to have it).

But this all begins to be nonsense. And so I found myself trying to put these disparate senses into a pattern, ordering them in an attempt to come to terms with them (an ineradicable habit inculcated by a medical education).

In the hierarchy, vision is leader. Great Art involves the sight: painting, architecture and fine vistas are the realm of the eye, the domain of princes. With its capacity to glean information from the farthest source, the eye is the most powerful. Pictures predominate over words: a clip of film says more than an intelligent description. The man-in-the-street, who has turned into the man-in-the-surgery, fears more the loss of sight than any other sense . . .

Close behind comes hearing – gateway to music and speech. Second only to a sight in gathering information from a distance, the sense of hearing also shares a nobility: the blithe spirit is extolled because of her soaring and singing.

But touch, smell and taste are definite poor relations. These are the more 'close at hand' senses. Even here, there is a pecking order. Touch has a fine classical – statuesque and erotic (hard and soft?) – tradition. Taste is swallowed down with quaffs of fine wine and culinary verbiage. But who goes on about smell? Smell has, shall we say, a bad aura. We smell a rat. An offence, being rank, 'smells to heaven'. Noses are screwed up when smells are spoken of. But smell can be very powerful – it need not be confined to the near. The salmon navigates huge distances by smell, homing in with his ancient brain. And a horse 'smelleth the battle afar off'

(Job 29.25). The sense of smell can have power over time as
well as distance with highly-sensed French novelists being
transported back into boyhood by a whiff . . .

Actually, I'm unconvinced that smell is as important in
traditional diagnostic medicine as is sometimes claimed. I will
never diagnose typhoid by the smell of 'freshly baked brown
bread', phenylketonuria by its alleged musty odour (said to
resemble stale locker-room towels − I prefer the bread, I
think) nor maple syrup urine disease by the smell of −
you've guessed it, maple syrup urine. And as for the oast-
house syndrome which describes the flaccid mentally
defective infant with hyperaminoaciduria smelling of dried
malt or hops . . .

But as a adjunct to general practice, an illustration of the
already known and a powerful reinforcer, it is not to be
underestimated. The obvious reminder that a patient smokes
or drinks is well known, as is the distinctive pong of melaena
− (I definitely prefer freshly baked brown bread smells,
whatever their source) − once smelled, never forgotten.
More subtly, smell gives extra colour (so to speak) to our
perception of our patients who of course do smell of many
things, such as their occupation. There are agricultural
aromas (sheep dip, disinfectants), that fine oily smell which
imbues workers from our local engineering factory and the
scents of the bath cubes from the ladies who spend all day
packing them.

Scents (indistinguishable, interestingly, from sense, when
spoken) are smells manipulated: they say a lot about their
owners − if not what they are, at least what they'd like to be
taken for. And some smells (or are they scents?) are
insensible, if you see what I mean − or should I say follow
my trail? − for now we read about pheromones (we might
hear about them or possibly even smell them). Messages in
smell, a language not yet described let alone understood, are
part of the vocabulary of non-verbal communication.

As sense extends, widens, dissolves and disappears into (I
am tempted to say abscence) what? − I am left with the
bewilderment of one who has failed and encountered the
senseless. I am left contemplating my ubiquitous and
increasingly omniscient companion which is nonetheless
insensate, the computer. It exists parasitically off my own

senses. Even when they come of age – which overstretches my senses – as with Hal in 2001, they will aspire only to the first two senses. Perhaps touch – the Army already has robot bomb-dismantling machines. And taste maybe: I hear that wines can be automatically assessed by computer.

But never smell. Whether it be newly-cut grass, the formalin-tinged air of the dissecting room, the cool smell of canvas when camping or freshly baked brown bread (the real thing, I mean) . . . of all the senses – whether they be five, seven or legion – one will always remain irrational, untamed, unfathomable in the deep brain's core and supremely sensitive.

RICHARD WESTCOTT
South Molton

World of Neurology

In the arcane world of neurology, nervous laughter sometimes represents recognition as much as amusement. I have a relationship with a nervous disease which dogs me, snaps unexpectedly at my heels and all but brings me down. Nervous laughter – mine – usually concludes the episode: the relief of recognition coupled with the ironic reflection that it will happen again. A good enough reason to laugh!

Thus, Linda – a big, cascading mother of two – presented with a muddled story of pain in the back. An infrequent attender with no history of back problems and no trauma, she was quite normal at examination: spine and movements undeniably normal, breath sounds unremarkable and try as I might I could hear no pleural rub, see any skin lesion, find any calf tenderness or pyrexia.

Believing in natural cures, she started on the virtues of yarrow and the comforts of camomile. I listened, trusting to some inner rumination to regurgitate a solution (it does happen, well, just occasionally). The balm of basil was being extolled when I surfaced as uninspired as at the outset. Her pain was real enough. Fortunately extroverts don't always insist on their doctor explaining everything. She swept out, helped not at all by me. Several days later, she returned triumphantly with the announcement that I might consider cider vinegar for my other patients with shingles. She was sure the straggly progress of those dreaded speckles had been brought up short by her own treatment. Another nervous laugh.

It's not just across the age range that shingles scatters its vesicles – it can appear, sinisterly from within, anywhere. Like a guerilla it strikes when and where least expected: the silent shingles, having slept awhile, slides down a nerve painlessly to burn on its emergence. Worse, and even more unsportsmanlike, its invisible pain precedes any stigma. More even than the wily spirochaete, this chameleon can take on many colours. Give me a good red-blooded disease with proper, recognizable signs and symptoms, predictable battle areas and individual character!

Slippery Zoster (Tolkien could not have found a better name) continues to fox with its underground terrorist tactics: it persists with unchivalrous behaviour and skilful sleight of hand in sliding from my mind. But once the villain is spotted – forgive the pun – I laugh. Nervously.

RICHARD WESTCOTT
South Molton

Piercing Pam's Ears

'O I'll do it for you,' I said impetuously, 'and it won't cost you a penny.' Student Nurse Pam Guest had set her heart on having pierced ears but pleaded poverty at the price. As a young houseman I cut a dash in my white coat; indeed I was utterly ignorant of all moral fear. There was nothing I would not undertake: a tracheostomy before breakfast, a trephine over lunch, a transplant after tea – I was perfectly imperturbable. So when pretty Pam Guest wanted pierced ears, but didn't have the £10 fee, I charged to the rescue. A modern-day Sir Lancelot, piercing ears and breaking hearts. 'It won't take a minute, Pam,' I said, sweeping aside all objections. We found a quiet corner in the sluice – not the most sterile surroundings I admit – but a chap has to start somewhere on the road to Harley Street. The sluice was at least out of harm's way, if not exactly a private consulting room.

I was quite disdainful of germs. My patients never had wound infections – microbes withered beneath my healing hands – and yet Pam would insist on cleaning her ears with a soapy antiseptic (the smell of which, even now, makes me quiver). I sat her down on the commode and stood behind her – a clever touch this, not letting her see the operation. 'What are you going to use?' she said. 'Oh, I've got an assortment of needles,' I replied casually, 'I don't think we need to raid theatre.' 'Aren't you going to freeze the skin?' Pam was having second thoughts. 'Now don't be soft love, and be a brave soldier. Just think of all those sailors at the battle of Trafalgar. I'm not going to amputate your leg, though you might need a bullet to bite on,' I added with good humour. 'Right, here we go,' I said in a masterful voice, 'It will all be over in two seconds.'

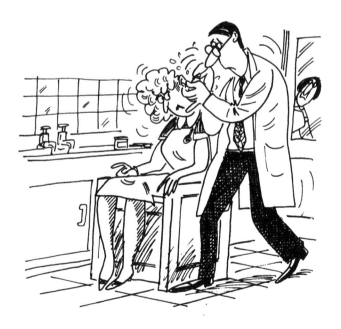

Have you ever tried to grab a soapy, slithery ear and push a needle through it?

This was an understatement. Have you ever tried to grab a soapy, slithery ear and push a needle through it? Amazingly difficult. Pam's lobe refused to stay still – it just wriggled about between my fingers. Imagine stabbing a jellied eel. And her skin was so tough. My own lobes feel as soft as kid gloves, but dear Pam's had the texture of elephant leather. I examined the needle – the point had bent over. 'I think I'll go to the shop after all,' said Pam, squirming on the commode. 'They use a gun there, and it's over before you can say . . . Ouch!' she screamed. 'That hurt!'

I had got the needle into the lobe but then realized that I could not push it right through without impaling my own fingers on the other side. Awkward. Blood was trickling down my fingers. I had not expected an arterial bleeder in such a dainty ear. I looked down at the patient: her face was green, and her white uniform was spatteredwith red drops. 'I think you'd better stop,' she wailed. 'But you can't have just one ear done,' I said in a quavering voice (this was before the era of the unilateral ear-ring). I turned to wipe my hands at the sink, and heard a dull thud. Pam had fallen forward from the commode, banging her head against the bath. She was out cold.

'Where has all the blood come from?' a voice shouted behind me. Staff Nurse Jones had come into the sluice with a bed-pan. 'Oh my God! Is she dead?' she said in a hushed voice. 'Of course not!' I shouted back. 'There's no need to panic.' I bent over the body. Only a faint, obviously. I felt her pulse beneath my trembling fingers. With my ear close to her mouth I could hear faint breathing.

As I was ministering to this fallen angel Sister Hughes, the ward tyrant, burst in behind Staff Nurse. 'Doctor Stocks!' she roared, 'What have you done to my nurse?' I looked down at poor Pam; I looked at the blood, my bloody hands, the dripping needle. What had I been up to? 'It's nothing Sister,' I laughed nervously, 'She's fainted, that's all.' 'Well don't give her the kiss of life whatever you do.' Sister turned on her heels and stormed out.

Within seconds the sluice was full of uninvited guests: nurses, porters and, worst of all, the crash-team. Pam groaned and opened her eyes. 'That's enough for one day,' she whispered. 'And that's quite enough of that!' said Staff Nurse, jumping to the wrong conclusion.

We were hospital gossip for weeks. The greatest calumny was that I was having my wicked way with a needle. The older nurses called me Van Gogh, and the younger ones gave me a wide berth on the corridor. But my consultant was very understanding.

'I'm sorry about the incident yesterday,' I murmured at the start of the ward-round. 'Oh that's all right,' he said, taking me to one side. 'Nurse Guest explained it all to Sister. She'll soon be out of sick-bay, and her ear hasn't turned septic – yet. Fortunately Sister keeps a very clean sluice. I did my first operation in the garden shed,' he added proudly, 'though the patient was a rag-doll of my sister's, not the living doll you found.' He seemed very pleased with his joke.

'I just wasn't expecting all that blood,' I said sheepishly. 'And the skin was so tough.' 'Well just remember young man, next time you nibble a nurse's ear don't bite off more than you can chew.'

DAVID STOCKS
Leeds

9 Administration

*W*here are the Matrons, the Sisters, the Lady Almoners of yesteryear? When I was a student, we had a Matron like a galleon in full sail; and Matron was what we called her. Then things went to the bad with the Salmon reorganization. I just can't get used to our present 'Patient Services Manager' – that's what Matron's have become – insisting on being called Ms Robinson, especially as he's a man!

The Health Service is riddled with gloom and despair. They are trying to run it like a grocer's shop but we trained to be doctors, not grocers. Even so, despite seven reorganizations in 19 years/19 reorganizations in seven years*, there are still occasional gleams of hope. As I told Mr William Waldegrave, our own hospital has managed to cut its waiting lists to one year. He said, 'Remind me, which is your hospital?' I told him, 'Queen Charlotte's Maternity Hospital.'

Paper in Health Service Maladministration

Attempt Six Questions

Question 1. 36 patients were referred to the Department of Medicine in a busy general hospital. Of these, 27 were marked urgent, three were marked malignant, one was marked routine and five were not marked. The medical staff at the hospital consisted of one consultant, one registrar and one SHO. The latter has been off sick pregnant since appointment.

Assuming each doctor can see three new patients each clinic, at three clinics per week, how long should a 25 year-old, unemployed man with a psychiatric history and a criminal record, complaining of a headache be expected to wait?

---

*Delete where appropriate.

(a) an unlimited time
(b) as long as possible
(c) he should be seen within the hour.
Comment on the long-term effects of these difficulties.

Question 2. A 15 year-old female has attempted suicide by gassing, wrist-cutting and overdosage five times in the last three months. It emerges from social investigations that her father, a company director with convictions for fraud, has been having an incestuous relationship with her, but denies it. Her father writes a letter of complaint to the District Administrator threatening to write to the local MP, the Department of Health and several other remote dignitaries to highlight the poor treatment he believes the girl has received at the local hospital, and by her general practitioner.

Write an essay on the role you would expect the police, the general practitioner, the social services, the gynaecologist, the venereologist, and the inland revenue, to play in the management of this case.

Question 3. In 1954, a small cottage hospital with 100 beds was administered by one hospital secretary assisted by a personal assistant. In 1983, the same hospital, with only 62 beds, was administered by one district administrator, four sector administrators, nine divisional administrators, five personal assistants, seven secretaries, and ten clerk assistants. Because of overspending, it is planned to cut five jobs but the various Unions, having got wind of this decision, are planning an all-out strike in an attempt to pre-empt it.

Of the various courses of action in your capacity as Minister of Health, would you:
(a) Close the hospital
(b) Sack all the administrators and appoint the first applicant from the job centre as Hospital Secretary
(c) Declare the area a nuclear-free zone, evacuate the patients and hand over the keys to the chairperson of the local lesbian revolutionary front.
Justify your decision to the next cabinet meeting.

Question 4. The local medical school dean is short of patients and as a consequence the academic staff are having to use

simulated patients. The academic staff committee offers ten honorary clinical demonstrator posts, plus a small remuneration, to local principals in general practice in exchange for free access to their lists. After several months all the partners demand a meeting with the principal. They explain that an increased work load has developed from having to reassure patients who have been overinvestigated, repeatedly admitted and prescribed large amounts of expensive medication. As principal should you:
(a) join a monastery
(b) take an overdose
(c) resign your clinical demonstratorship and emigrate
(d) write a paper on iatrogenic hypochondriasis.

Comment on the service role of ivory towers in the NHS in general.

Question 5. One of your partners in general practice requests an urgent meeting with you (the principal). Over a pint, your colleague describes an affliction of his testicles which concerns him greatly. You refer him to the local surgeon, who decides after a full examination and tests, including WR, that there is nothing physically wrong with him. Shortly after this, you are called to the surgery to find that the doctor had displayed his testicles to a female patient, declaring that the SDP had flashed electric pulses, via the National Grid, to his genitals and that the universe was on the brink of World War III.

Do you:
(a) bundle the poor soul into a van under the cover of darkness, and smuggle him in a drugged state on to a container vessel marked 'Livestock – Do Not Disturb'
(b) pretend that he is an escaped mental patient and mumble about not coming home on leave again
(c) lace his morning coffee with chlorpromazine and ask the local shrink to do a domiciliary visit.

Present a report to the GMC with a view to his reinstatement, assuming his mental state is unchanged after six months of in-patient treatment.

M. A. LAUNER
Burnley

Psychiatric Out-patients

Ten nervous patients, sitting in a line
One got taken short, and then there were nine.
Nine nervous patients, settled down to wait
One threw a wobbly, and then there were eight.
Eight nervous patients, booked in at eleven
One came an hour late, and then there were seven.
Seven nervous patients hoping for a 'fix'
One had a bad trip, and then there were six.
Six nervous patients, glad to be alive
One took a manic turn, and then there were five.
Five nervous patients, waiting near the door
One made a dash for it, and then there were four.
Four nervous patients, sent by their GP
One lost his doctor's note, and then there were three.
Three nervous patients, feeling rather blue
One took an overdose, and then there were two.
Two nervous patients started having fun
One became pregnant, and then there was one.
One nervous patient, treatment just begun
The hospital closed down, and then there were none.

MARIE CAMPKIN
London

Wednesday the Thirteenth

N ever mind what people say about Friday the Thirteenth.
Wednesday the Thirteenth can be pretty unpropitious as
well. The first patient in is Mrs Moscow. She is an Italian
married to a Ukrainian with a 23-year-old son who is
decidedly odd. Last night the son's oddness reached melt-
down and he went haywire. Would I call round?

Alfredo has smashed the television set, broken a light
fitting, and chased his sister round the house. He has heard
voices accusing him of having VD. I am no expert but it is
clear that, at this moment, Alfredo is to sanity what Jeffrey

Archer is to classical literature. I contact the duty psychiatrist who says, 'Leave it all to me.'

I am up a ladder excavating my guttering when the 'phone rings. The psychiatrist wants me at the patient's house *pronto* to sign the Section 2 form.

I arrive back at the house to find Alfredo throwing cups through the kitchen window. The psychiatrist has gone, leaving a social worker to arrange transport. We are in the middle of the ambulance dispute and she has had to contact the police. A policeman arrives and we evolve a plan to convey Alfredo to the hospital in the social worker's car with the strong arm of the law on one side and the trembling arm of the GP on the other.

Reinforcements arrive in the form of a police sergeant. By now, Alfredo is perched, like a parrot, on top of the sofa, and is treating the constable to a spectacular display of linguistic pyrotechnics, demonstrating his ability to swear in Italian, French, and Ukrainian, as well as English. For reasons not entirely apparent, the sergeant declares that Alfredo should be brought down from his perch and stretched out on the sofa. This escalates Alfredo's aggression and it is decided that he should be handcuffed. The police officers sit on him, while I grab the legs.

I suddenly realize that the limbs I am restraining are covered in dark blue serge. 'Thank you,' booms the sergeant as I hurriedly release them, 'I never knew you cared.'

It is becoming obvious that a car will prove an inadequate means of transport. A police van will be needed, and for that you need the authority of a police inspector. This worthy is duly summoned. He beams benignly at Alfredo, and says 'Well, lad, how're you doing?'

Alfredo responds with a well-aimed kick at the inspector's wedding tackle.

'Can't you give him something to quieten him down?' he grimaces. I rummage in my bag and produce 100 mg of intramuscular chlorpromazine.

Within ten minutes Alfredo is semi-comatose on the sofa. This provides a much-needed respite and heavy hints are dropped about the parched state of various throats. Mrs Moscow is encouraged into the kitchen where she busies herself with the cups that Alfredo has not thrown out of the window. In the meantime, the social worker has finally managed to summon a real ambulance and Alfredo goes as quietly as a lamb. It has been an interesting afternoon, but the next time the thirteeth falls on a Wednesday, I think I'll cut my losses and stay in bed.

LAURENCE KNOTT
Enfield

Index

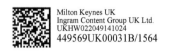

Milton Keynes UK
Ingram Content Group UK Ltd.
UKHW022049141024
449569UK00031B/1564

9 781870 905800